By the Editors of Consumer Guide®

MEDICAL BOOK OF REMEDIES:

50 Ways to

MANAGE DIABETES

In Association With
The American Association of Diabetes Educators
Jean Betschart M.N., R.N., C.D.E.

PUBLICATIONS INTERNATIONAL, LTD.

Author: Jean Betschart, M.N., R.N., C.D.E.
Consulting Organization: The American Association of Diabetes Educators
Coordinating Consultant: Susan Thom, R.D., L.D., C.H.E.
Consultants: Kris Ernst, R.N., C.H.E.
Karmeen Kulkarni, M.S., R.D., C.H.E.
Marilyn Graff, B.S.N., R.N., C.H.E.
Richard Rubin, Ph.D., C.H.E.
Deborah Hinnen Hentzen, M.N., R.N., C.H.E.
Illustrator: Yoshi Miyake

The American Association of Diabetes Educators (AADE) was established in 1974 and is a multidisciplinary organization dedicated to advancing the role of the diabetes educator and improving the quality of diabetes education and care. The organization is composed of more than 9,500 health care professionals, including nurses, dietitians, pharmacists, and physicians.

Jean Betschart is Diabetes Program Coordinator at Children's Hospital of Pittsburgh and adjunct faculty in the University of Pittsburgh Parent-Child Program. A past President of the American Association of Diabetes Educators, she was awarded the American Diabetes Association's Outstanding Health Professional Educator Award in 1994. She has published several books for children, adolescents, and adults, including *It's Time to Learn About Diabetes,* and she is a contributor to *Diabetes Self-Management.*

Susan Thom is a clinical specialist with Diabetes Associates, concentrating on diabetes counseling, weight management, and community education. She is the President of the American Association of Diabetes Educators. She is the media and resources spokesperson for the American Dietetic Association and serves on the board of directors of the Juvenile Diabetes Foundation's Cleveland Chapter and Ho Mita Koda camp, the first diabetes camp in the world.

Kris Ernst is a diabetes nurse educator and clinical education specialist at the Emory Clinic in Atlanta, where she is involved in individual and group instruction in diabetes self-management. President-Elect of the American Association of Diabetes Educators, she has held positions with the National Certification Board for Diabetes Education (NCBDE) and has held the presidency of the Greater Atlanta Association of Diabetes Educators.

Karmeen Kulkarni is the Director of Nutrition Services at the Diabetes Health Center in Salt Lake City. Her areas of specialty include diabetes education, weight management, and diabetes team management. She serves as Vice President of the American Association of Diabetes Educators.

Marilyn Graff is coordinator of Longmont Clinic in Colorado. A diabetes education consultant at medical offices in Boulder, Denver, and Longmont, she has been educating health care professionals and people with diabetes for 14 years. She serves as Secretary of the American Association of Diabetes Educators.

Richard Rubin is a part-time instructor at Johns Hopkins University School of Medicine and partner at Diabetes Consultation Services, a private practice in Baltimore devoted to people with diabetes and their families. He serves as Treasurer of the American Association of Diabetes Educators and President of the Maryland affiliate of the American Diabetes Association, and he is co-author of *Psyching Out Diabetes.*

Deborah Hinnen Hentzen is program director of the Diabetes Treatment and Research Center at St. Joseph Medical Center in Wichita, Kansas. She is a past President of the American Association of Diabetes Educators, associate editor of *A Core Curriculum for Diabetes Education,* and past chair of the AADE Continuing Education Committee. She also served as the national chair of the American Diabetes Association education council and was honored as the National Diabetes Educator of the Year by the AADE in 1986.

8 7 6 5 4 3 2 1

ISBN: 0-7853-1233-1

CONTENTS

C O N T E N T S

INTRODUCTION

Managing diabetes can be frustrating, challenging, and rewarding. Diabetes impacts every aspect of life from food preparation and eating to family planning and intimacy. It affects personal interactions and it can impact work situations.

Fitting diabetes into a life full of other responsibilities and priorities always seems to require a twist, a turn, or a compromise. It's true that balancing control of blood glucose levels with other physical, emotional, or social priorities requires a lot of energy. Indeed, the word "control" smacks of full-time effort. But you can manage diabetes without completely disrupting your life. The idea is for you to control diabetes so it doesn't control you. This book shows you how to fit diabetes management into your life more easily while you achieve the very best level of control you can.

One of the important lessons of this book is that you are not alone—no matter what your current level of control or what type of diabetes you have. About 85 percent of people with diabetes have Type II (non–insulin-dependent) diabetes. Most of these people are older than 40 years of age and overweight; often they have a strong family history of diabetes. They manage diabetes with diet and exercise and perhaps an oral agent—a pill to help regulate blood glucose levels. Type II diabetes is a disease of insulin resistance: The insulin present is ineffective or unable to reach the body's muscle and fat cells. Occasionally, those with Type II diabetes may require insulin injections if the disease is not otherwise well controlled.

People with Type I diabetes are usually young and of normal weight. Type I diabetes is an autoimmune disease, which means the body makes antibodies (infection-fighting cells) against itself. The antibodies destroy the cells that make insulin (beta cells); therefore, no more insulin is made. People with this type of disease require injections of insulin to make up for the insulin the body does not make.

Why is diabetes management so important? People with diabetes have an increased risk of developing other serious medical conditions such as retinopathy (disorders of the retina of the eye), nephropathy (kidney disease), and neuropathy (disease involving the nerves). Studies have shown that reducing your average blood glucose level can significantly reduce the risk of these diabetes-related conditions. One of the largest of these studies, the Diabetes Control and Complications Trial (DCCT), was completed in 1993. DCCT followed 1,400 people with Type I diabetes, aged 13 to 39 years. The study participants were divided into two groups based on the type of care: The first group received standard diabetes care; the other received "intensive management." Intensive management consisted of four injections of insulin per day, an insulin pump, nutrition counseling, and behavioral support to try to maintain blood glucose levels at more normal levels. DCCT found that the subjects who kept their blood glucose levels as close to normal as possible had a 60 percent reduction in their risk of development and progression of eye, kidney, and nervous system complications.

This book describes some of the ways you can bring your blood glucose levels closer to normal. It is important to work with your physician, diabetes educator, or other health care professional to plan a diabetes management program. Don't hesitate to ask these professionals questions or seek their counsel about incorporating the advice in this book into your management program. Also ask them to provide you with materials about DCCT. Remember that diabetes care must be individualized; you may need to try a variety of suggestions and techniques to find those that work best for you. The reward for your diligence is feeling healthy and in control.

50 Ways to Manage Diabetes contains general tips for all people with diabetes as well as a section for those who use insulin. The first section of the book proposes what you need to begin a program of diabetes self-management: a positive outlook, the determination to succeed, a qualified health care team, and a strong support network in friends and family. Section two describes the equipment you'll need to successfully manage diabetes. The third section provides advice on meal planning and explains the recent guidelines of the American Diabetes Association. The next section explains how to prevent diabetes-related medical conditions. Section five is devoted to suggestions for those who require insulin to manage diabetes, and the final section offers tips to stay motivated in your diabetes care and energized in your life—to stay active, stay healthy, and live your life to the fullest.

DECIDE TO DO IT.

Most of the time, we have a pretty good idea what we should do to maintain our health and well-being. The hard part is actually doing it. We're familiar with the drill: Brush and floss our teeth, exercise regularly, reduce fat and cholesterol, reduce stress, limit alcohol intake, see the doctor for checkups. But how many of us consistently perform these healthy habits? The answer is, very few! So it's no surprise that it is equally—if not more—difficult to manage diabetes consistently.

We know the tasks persons with diabetes must perform: take medication, test blood glucose levels, follow a prescribed meal plan, exercise regularly, and keep accurate and current records. Doing it all is tough! And it's especially hard if we think we may need to perform these tasks for the rest of our lives. So why keep up with them at all?

Research has proved that control of blood glucose levels can decrease markedly the risk of diabetes-related complications such as blindness and kidney disease in people with insulin-dependent diabetes. It can also slow their advance in people who already have signs of these conditions. Therefore, experts believe all people with diabetes should manage their blood glucose levels to protect their future health and well-being and live a long, healthy, productive life.

The problem for most people seems to be waiting for the motivation "on/off" switch in the brain to click "on." Experts know a person must go through a certain readiness period before starting a new behavior. Some people take a long time to get ready; others do it fairly quickly. The amount of time it takes depends on how many obstacles litter the way and how much support is available to help overcome those obstacles.

Since you're reading this book, perhaps you are nearly ready to click to "on." You've decided to recruit the help you need to remove the obstacles and fit diabetes into your life. Remember, diabetes control doesn't happen overnight. It's a process—and you won't be perfect at it every day. But, as this book reminds you, you won't be alone either. Others have been successful—you can be, too.

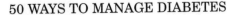

2 | FIT DIABETES INTO YOUR LIFE!

Let's be honest. It's not easy to fit diabetes into your life without making it the center of your existence. The people who accomplish this seem to perform their diabetes tasks quietly, not making a big deal about them. They test their blood glucose routinely, adjusting their meals, activity, or diabetes medication according to their schedule. They have learned to work diabetes into their lifestyle. To them, diabetes care comes as naturally as brushing their teeth each morning. If you're having trouble getting on track with diabetes management, try these tips:

- Stock the proper tools. Keep plenty of diabetes supplies, such as lancets, testing strips for blood and urine, diabetes medication, syringes, and glucose tablets or juice, on hand. Make sure you have replacement batteries for your glucose meter and an extra pen for recording your blood glucose results. A travel or cosmetics case can keep supplies together, organized, and portable. Consider having two meters, one at home and one at work for easy access.

- Purchase appropriate foods to make diabetes care easy for you. If you must buy desserts and other temptations for your family, store them out of sight. Temptation that stares you in the face is hard to resist.

- If you find yourself in a slump with your care, enlist the support of family and friends to remind you to keep up with your testing and medication. Bear in mind your testing does not become their responsibility; it is yours.

- Devise ways to remind yourself. Leave your meter in an obvious location so you remember to test. Leave yourself notes in conspicuous places. Synchronize the testing and/or medication to coincide with other activities in your daily routine; for example, when the coffee is brewing in the morning, test your blood glucose.

- Establish a routine. It sounds so obvious, but if you establish a routine for your care, diabetes management becomes an automatic response, even when you feel stressed or pressured by other events in your life.

- Don't let diabetes care keep you from doing something you really want to do. With frequent testing and a good understanding of your diabetes care, you can participate in most activities you enjoy.

People who are successful at diabetes control have learned to be good problem solvers. This is a skill that takes practice. It's important that you work at developing your problem-solving skills.

Start by defining the problem and identifying the barriers to solving it. Be as specific as you can. Perhaps you fall off your program in the hectic hours of dinner time. You and your spouse have just arrived home from work; you've picked the kids up from various points: day care, soccer practice, the library. Everyone's hungry and a little tired; you had a bad day at work, and you're tired and cranky yourself. You want to hear about everyone's day, but they're all talking at once. You need to eat but dinner won't be ready for a while yet, so you grab the first item you see in the refrigerator. Then you realize you forgot to take your diabetes medication.

In this scenario, the problem is staying in good control around dinner time. The barriers to overcoming the problem are everyone's different, hectic schedules. Once you identify the problems and barriers, you find resources to deal with them. Keep healthy snack foods on hand—cut-up carrots and celery, apples, granola bars—to tide everyone over until dinner is on the table. Arrange for younger children to get a snack before you pick them up from day care. Older kids can pack a snack to take with them to school, and you can pack a snack to eat before you leave work. You and your spouse can prepare and freeze some meals ahead of time for quick preparation. Perhaps you need to work on some stress busters so you don't come home from work so wound up (see Remedy 31). Take a walk with your kids before or after dinner to hear about their day.

Do you see how this works? When you confront problems, you realize you have options to solve them. You will feel less manipulated and more in control of yourself and your future. If you find the solutions to your problems are not as simple as those outlined here, you may need to get help from books, classes, or a counselor or diabetes educator. Do whatever it takes!

3 ASSEMBLE A WINNING TEAM.

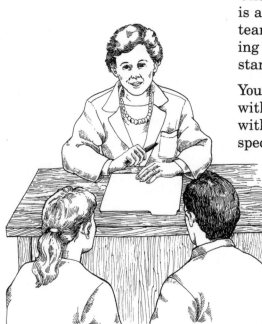

One of the most important elements of a successful diabetes care program is a health care provider. Whether you work with one professional or a team of professionals, you should feel your health care provider is willing to listen to your concerns and take the time to make sure you understand how best to manage diabetes.

Your doctor may be an endocrinologist, a doctor who specializes in dealing with hormonal problems. (Insulin is a hormone.) A child or adolescent with diabetes may be cared for by a pediatric endocrinologist who has special knowledge about diabetes in children. If an endocrinologist is not available in your area, choose a doctor who has experience in diabetes care. Ultimately, a physician's most important qualification is that you feel comfortable with him or her.

Ideally, a multidisciplinary team is available to you. The team may include a doctor, nurse educator, registered dietitian, social worker, psychologist or psychiatrist, and exercise physiologist. But all of these specialists may not be available in the area in which you live or the health care setting you use. You and your doctor may need to put together your own team:

• Ask your doctor to refer you to a diabetes educator or dietitian. The American Association of Diabetes Educators can also provide you with names; phone them at 1-800-TEAMUP4 (832-6874).

• Look for professionals with the credential C.D.E, which stands for Certified Diabetes Educator. This abbreviation assures you this licensed provider has met certain education requirements and has passed an examination that verifies knowledge and expertise in diabetes.

Finding a health care professional who is sensitive to your needs and able to provide the support you need is critical to your diabetes care. Communication is vital: Are you comfortable talking with this person? Is he or she readily available and willing to take time to answer questions or help with medication adjustments? You may need to talk with a few health care professionals before you find one who is right for you.

TAKE THE HELM.

4

The formation of diabetes care teams as described in Remedy 3 marks a shift in diabetes care. Traditionally, a doctor would tell you what to do, and you were expected to go home and do it. But with health care systems changing, people must learn to be advocates for themselves. The doctor is no longer the center of the team. You're in the driver's seat; it is up to you to steer the direction of your care. If you're unsure how to be an advocate for yourself, here are a few suggestions:

- Don't settle for someone who will not work with you to keep diabetes under optimal control. If a health care provider is too busy to spend time with you or seems unaware of how best to help you, find someone else. Even if you've been seeing one physician for a long time, do not feel compelled to stick with him or her. Place *your* needs first. A physician who is unable to help you because of patient load or lack of experience with diabetes is not the best physician for you, no matter how long you've known him or her.

- Ask your physician to refer you to a diabetes educator, registered dietitian, and/or psychologist if you have difficulty in areas where these professionals can help. And don't feel put out or dismissed if your physician refers you to one of these professionals without your asking. A physician who recognizes that others can help where he or she cannot is putting your needs first.

- Tell your health care provider what part of your management program you can do easily and where you have difficulty. Together you can come up with ideas to smooth the rocky areas and reinforce the already-strong areas. Also see Remedy 2 for advice on problem solving.

- Stay abreast of new research and developments in diabetes care (see Remedy 6 for more information). Ask your health care provider if new products might benefit you.

- Demand frequent communication with your health care provider so he or she can carefully monitor your blood glucose levels.

5 DEVELOP A POSITIVE OUTLOOK.

Successful diabetes control requires a positive outlook. That's a simple statement, but it's a significant point. You must think that controlling diabetes is a worthwhile endeavor, or you won't do it. And if you don't believe you will ever succeed, you probably won't. How do you forge a positive attitude? Start by recognizing that you can take steps to alter your health.

- Decide to make the best of it. You can't change the fact you have diabetes, so your choices are either to deny and ignore it or accept it and deal with it.

- Find something bigger than yourself to believe in. Free yourself from focusing on and constantly worrying about your own problems and concerns. Join a charitable organization, church group, or advocacy group. Become a hospital volunteer or a Big Brother or Sister.

- Practice visualization. Close your eyes and see yourself as healthy, active, and in good control of diabetes.

- Make an effort to find the positives both in life and in diabetes. Managing diabetes may give you more of a sense of control of your fate. Quitting smoking can help you feel more disciplined. Weight loss can boost your self-esteem. Joining an exercise program can lead to new friends. Make a list of positive elements, and review it on down days.

- Enlist the help of family and friends to keep you motivated. Avoid negative people who make you feel sad or bad about yourself. Surround yourself with people who care about you and will help you with the many tasks that are part of diabetes control.

- Reward yourself for jobs well done, such as when you lose five pounds or keep excellent records for a week.

- Understand that you will experience ups and downs. You will follow your regimen better at some times than you will at others. Don't be too hard on yourself or make excuses when you fall off your program. Admit you slipped, then try to determine why so you can prevent another fall.

BE A SPONGE!

6

Soak up as much diabetes information as you can hold! The more you know about diabetes, the better prepared you will be to handle problems if they crop up. Some people attempt to cope by denying their diabetes and its harmful effects. But this head-in-the-sand approach leaves them unable to deal with the trials and frustrations of diabetes management. In most cases, you are the only one who can make decisions about your care on a daily basis. Your doctor, diabetes educator, or registered dietitian cannot be with you 24 hours a day. The more you know, the better the decisions you will make.

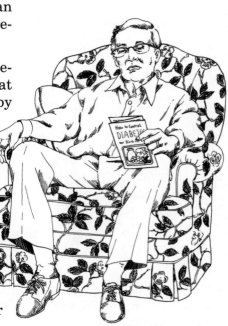

- Read as much as you can about diabetes. Ask your educator for materials and sources. Many publications about diabetes are available at your local library. You can also subscribe to newsletters published by manufacturers of glucose meters.

- Join the American Diabetes Association (ADA) and/or the Juvenile Diabetes Foundation International (JDFI). Call the ADA at 1-800-232-3472 and the JDFI at 1-800-223-1138 for more information.

- Stay abreast of new research technologies through publications and your diabetes educator.

- Call the ADA's Diabetes Information and Action Line (DIAL) at 1-800-351-5800 if you have any questions related to diabetes or would like referrals to ADA programs and community resources.

- Understand the importance of controlling diabetes. If you are unclear about any aspect, talk to your health care professional.

- Attend classes or seminars on diabetes given by a local hospital or the ADA or JDFI.

- Talk to others about how they care for their diabetes. Find out what works for them. You can do this by joining a support group run by the ADA, JDFI, or a local hospital.

- Ask questions of knowledgeable people: doctors, nurses, pharmacists, registered dietitians, and so on.

7

MAKE IT A FAMILY AFFAIR.

TEACH YOUR FAMILY:

- What diabetes is
- The types of diabetes
- How diabetes is treated
- Your individual treatment plan
- The importance of meal planning, preparation, and timing
- About your medications (how to inject insulin, if appropriate)
- The signs of hypoglycemia
- The treatment for hypoglycemia and where you keep supplies
- Your plan of record keeping
- How to help with sick days
- Emergency phone numbers

Diabetes is called a family disease because it affects every family member. Food selection and preparation as well as the timing of meals are important aspects of family life. The need for medication and avoidance of hypoglycemia (low blood glucose) can take away some spontaneity from meals. Dining out presents a whole new challenge.

Your diabetes management affects your family in other ways, too. They undoubtedly have feelings about your health, ranging from concern and sympathy to guilt and resentment. They may also worry about their own susceptibility to diabetes. Perhaps your treatment affects your family financially. Perhaps you require your family's help to pick up (or even administer) your medication or drive you to appointments with your doctor or diabetes educator. Recognize that the more your family members know about diabetes control, the more you all benefit. To get your family involved:

- Ask family members to attend diabetes education classes with you. Their direct participation involves them more effectively than your simply explaining what was taught, and they have the opportunity to ask questions of the instructor. Discuss what each of you learned, and ask your educator to clarify any discrepancies.

- Provide your family with reading materials. Encourage them to join the American Diabetes Association.

- Practice skills at home with your family: Perform finger sticks for blood glucose, inject saline into an orange or doll, and review the treatment for hypoglycemia so family members can understand what you go through and also carry out these acts in case of emergency.

- Make sure family members know your meal and medication schedule. Tell them how you plan to handle any schedule changes so they're prepared in the event of complications.

- Encourage any family member who is having trouble coping with your having diabetes to seek counseling to discuss his or her feelings.

TEACH YOUR FRIENDS.

Some people are reluctant to tell others about their diabetes care needs. But friends who care can help you stay on top of your program. Friends will take their attitude about diabetes from you. If you see it as a stigma, they may be reluctant to help you. On the other hand, if they see you taking charge of your condition and talking about it openly and honestly, they will feel more confident about helping you remain in control.

Friends won't know how they can support you unless you tell them. Here are ways to help your friends understand the role of diabetes in your life:

- Let others know how they can help you: "It really helps me when I see you order healthy foods off the menu first. . . ." Let them know how you feel about them eating sweet foods and desserts in front of you. Some people find it difficult to not eat what everyone else has; others don't mind at all when their friends have sweet foods. Clear the air with your friends, and cast off everyone's uncertainty about what to do.

- Encourage your friends to jump on the bandwagon. Everyone can—and should—eat a low-fat, well-balanced diet. Explain that just because you have diabetes, you needn't eat foods that are "different" from what everyone else is eating. The healthful behaviors you adopt to control diabetes and your weight are elements of a healthy lifestyle everyone can participate in.

- Prompt a friend to join you in an exercise or weight control program.

- Describe the signs and symptoms of hypoglycemia (low blood glucose) and how to treat it. Show friends where you keep treatment supplies, such as glucose tablets, juice, candy, or a Glucagon emergency kit, and explain how much of each you should receive in the event you do not recognize the signs yourself.

- Show friends where you carry your emergency phone numbers. Keep a list posted near your phone so visitors can find the numbers easily.

- Engage your friends in diabetes-related activities through the ADA or JDFI. Ask your friends to participate in a fund-raiser walk with you.

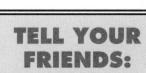

TELL YOUR FRIENDS:

- The signs and symptoms of hypoglycemia

- How you treat hypoglycemia

- Where you keep supplies

- Emergency phone numbers

- How you plan to manage meals, diabetes medication, and so forth around special events

- The importance of eating on time

- Other ways you would like them to participate in your diabetes management

9 GEAR UP!

A variety of supplies are available to help you care for diabetes. Most likely, you will choose your equipment based on the recommendations of your physician or educator, the cost, and your personal preferences. If your local drugstore does not carry the diabetes supplies you need or want, ask your pharmacist to order them. You can also order equipment and supplies by mail. Let's take a look at some of the supplies you need:

Meters to Measure Blood Glucose Levels

Ask your diabetes educator to recommend a meter appropriate for your needs. Most meters last three to four years. Prices will vary (from $10 to $100) as will their individual features. Consider buying two meters if you are on the go a lot—one for home and one for your purse, briefcase, backpack, or desk. Before you purchase a meter, consider the following:

- Do you need a meter with a memory? Some meters store the date, time, and result of previous blood glucose tests; some also give your average blood glucose level. Some meters have no memory.

  - How quickly do you need results? Depending on the meter, it can take from 20 seconds to 2 minutes to obtain results.

  - How do you maintain the meter? Is cleaning necessary? How difficult is it to clean?

  - How many steps does testing require; that is, do you need to do timing, wiping, or other additional steps that make testing complicated?

- Will the meter tell you when something is wrong—not enough blood, a dirty window, poor timing? Can it still yield accurate results despite some minor imperfections in your testing technique?

- Is it easy to calibrate the meter to the type of testing strips you have?

- What kind of batteries (if any) does it have? How often do they need to be replaced? (Generally, batteries should be good for at least 1,000 tests.)

- How large is the meter? Can you carry it in a pocket or purse?

- Does the manufacturer provide technical support in case you have a problem with the meter? Does the manufacturer have an 800 number for customer service?

- What is the cost of the strips the meter uses? (Your doctor or educator may recommend generic strips.)

Lancets to Obtain Blood for Testing

Lancets vary according to the size of the point and the depth of penetration. Some are designed for children or people with especially sensitive fingers.

- Ask your diabetes educator to give you a variety of lancets to sample. All meters come with finger-prick devices, and you can use most lancets with most devices.

- If you use a lancing device, check to see if its end-cap (the end that covers the lancet) has holes of different diameters to let the lancet through. This features allows you to adjust the end-cap for calloused fingers so you can obtain a deeper puncture and thus a better blood sample.

Remember: Never share your finger-pricking device without first cleaning the end-cap with a bleach solution. End-caps can transmit blood-borne viruses such as hepatitis or human immunodeficiency virus (HIV), the virus that causes AIDS. And *never* share lancets.

Syringes to Inject Insulin

The size of the syringe you use depends on your maximum dose of insulin. Insulin is measured in units. Insulin syringes come in 25, 30, 50, and 100 unit sizes. The needles for each are the same size; the numbers correspond to the size of the barrel of the syringe. When purchasing syringes, allow about 15 percent extra space in the event you need to increase your dose of insulin. If your usual dose is 50 units, buy 100-unit syringes so you're prepared if your doctor increases your dose to, say, 53 units.

Many people safely reuse their insulin syringes. After an injection, they simply recap the syringe and store it with their insulin. Do not do this if there is any chance someone else might be stuck with the needle. However, if you require two or three injections a day, you can use one syringe for the day and then discard it.

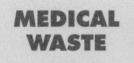

MEDICAL WASTE

Be sure to follow this advice for handling used equipment:

- Dispose of your syringes and lancets in a tightly capped, well-labeled container.

- Call your township, city, or borough for information regarding disposal of medical waste in your area.

PUT TWO AND TWO TOGETHER.

Until it becomes second nature, you must think about how diabetes medication, food, exercise, stress, illness, and other variables all work together to affect your blood glucose level. Understanding the balance can be complex, but it is vital to your diabetes management skills to do so. And even once you understand and incorporate the balance, you may be frustrated to find your glucose levels are still not where you want them to be.

Here are some factors that may cause blood glucose levels to rise and fall.

Makes Glucose Levels Go Up	**Makes Glucose Levels Go Down**
Food	Missed, delayed, or inadequate meal
Stress	Exercise
Not enough medication	Diabetes medication

Every element in one column corresponds with an element in the other. For example, exercise lowers blood glucose levels, so one way to balance the level is to eat more.

The type of insulin you take also plays a significant role. Insulin has a peak action time—the time it has its strongest effect on your blood glucose levels. Each kind of insulin works differently. See Remedy 37 for peak action times of different types of insulin. To keep track of all the factors that contribute to diabetes control:

- Test your blood glucose before and after you eat or exercise more than usual, and record any impact.

- Track how your blood glucose level responds to different foods. For example, see how the level increases after you eat similar amounts of potatoes, pasta, or corn. Do the same with similar foods: Compare sugar-sweetened cereals with those containing relatively little sugar.

- Highlight high or low blood glucose levels on your record sheets in different colors (see Remedy 42). See if high or low blood glucose values correspond to the peak action times of insulin(s).

- Share the information from frequent testing with your health professional so together you can fine-tune your management.

STICK TO A ROUTINE.

One of the most helpful strategies to control blood glucose levels is sticking to a schedule. Granted, it isn't always easy to stick to a routine in our busy lives, but there are many reasons to try. First, maintaining a consistent schedule of eating, exercise, and use of medication helps to identify patterns of highs and lows in your blood glucose records so you can adjust your program for better control.

If you have Type II diabetes and diet and exercise are your means of diabetes control, it is less important for you to follow a schedule rigidly. Or if you use an insulin pump or a multiple daily injection plan (three or more injections a day), you may already have more flexibility in your schedule (see Remedy 39).

Try these techniques for creating a feasible schedule:

- Write down your normal daily routine. With your diabetes educator's help, identify changes that could help you obtain better control. For example, if you notice your blood glucose runs too low on days you play tennis, you may need to reduce your medication or eat more on those days.

- Establish a daily exercise time, whether morning, afternoon, or evening. Many people find they have the most energy and get the most out of exercise when they exercise early in the morning. In addition, blood glucose does not fall quite as easily in response to morning exercise. If you have Type I diabetes, you may need to exercise after breakfast to ensure that your blood glucose doesn't drop too low.

- If you know your schedule will change for a week or even a day and you're unsure how to fit diabetes management in, consult your educator or doctor. For example, your child's soccer game or that pro basketball game you finally got tickets for may overlap with the supper hour; you're attending an afternoon wedding and the meal will be served at 3 P.M.; or your family is gathering for Mother's Day brunch at 10 A.M.

With a little strategizing, these schedule shifts can fit in smoothly. For more tips on handling special occasions, see Remedy 24.

- Try to stay within 1 to 1½ hours of your regular schedule.

- Try to wake about the same time every day—even on weekends. If you get up at 6:30 during the week and 10:30 on weekends, you may wake on those late mornings with a blood glucose level that is too high or too low. Also, because you're starting your day later than usual, you're likely to throw off all your meal times or end up compressing your meals into a shorter overall period. As Remedy 10 discusses, diabetes control requires a balance. When you make a change in one area, such as in your schedule or in amounts of food or exercise, you may need to adjust one of the other elements. What you adjust is up to you; there are no rules. If sleeping late causes a pattern of high blood glucose at lunch, you could: 1) eat less at breakfast; 2) eat lunch later; 3) increase Regular insulin in the morning; 4) exercise in the morning. Or you may need to select a combination of these approaches. Be sure to cover the peak times of your medications with a snack. And don't give yourself the next shot until the medication you took previously has peaked.

- If you want to change your regular schedule for some reason, such as a vacation, alter your schedule gradually, testing your blood glucose level frequently. Try moving your morning diabetes medication and breakfast a half hour later each day until you get on your new schedule. Again, look for a pattern of high or low blood glucose over three or four days. If a pattern develops, you may need to adjust food, medication, exercise, or your schedule.

- Try to keep food quantities and types of foods consistent. The greater the consistency, the better you can predict how your blood glucose will respond.

- Develop a pattern for insulin injections. For example, take all injections in your abdomen. Or take morning injections in your arms, evening injections in your legs. This technique helps cut down on variability of insulin absorption that can occur when you use different sites.

TEST WITHOUT FAIL.

Testing your blood glucose levels is your most valuable tool to determine how successful you are at diabetes control. And thanks to current technology, testing is easy. True, most people will never enjoy poking their finger for a drop of blood, but the new lancets make this step more comfortable, and the newest meters, which are small, portable, convenient, and fast, can make the rest of the testing process absolutely painless.

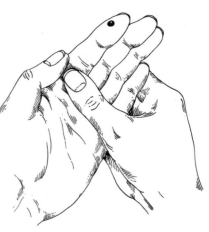

Tips for Performing the Finger Stick

Still make a face every time you do a finger stick? Believe it or not, you will get used to it. Rotate fingers. Experiment with sites. And follow these tips to smooth and uniform finger sticks.

- Wash your hands. Clean fingers reduce the risk of infection, but cleanliness also ensures accuracy of test results. Soap and water is fine for cleansing. Alcohol in single-use packets is a good choice when soap and water are not handy but not a good choice for everyday use. Alcohol can dry the skin and, if not wiped away, can cause a false-high reading when it mixes with blood. Dry your hands thoroughly.

- Warm your hands to increase blood supply to the area. Hang them down, shake them, or wash them in warm water. Milk the finger from the base to the tip to increase blood flow to the fingertip.

- Anchor your finger on a tabletop. You'll be less likely to get a stick that is too shallow.

- Use the sides of your fingers and thumbs. These areas are less sensitive and rich in capillary blood.

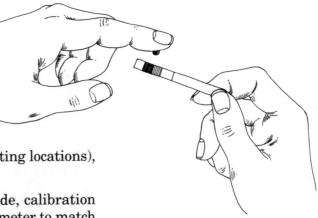

Tips for Meter Use

Once you've selected a meter suitable for your needs (see Remedy 9), follow this advice.

- Keep lancets, alcohol (if necessary for out-of-the-way testing locations), testing strips, and your record sheet together.

- Check your meter's accuracy frequently. Change the code, calibration chip, or strip when appropriate. (You need to adjust your meter to match each bottle or box of strips you use.) The meter comes with instructions to perform this simple procedure.

When to Test Blood Glucose

When you test depends on your doctor's recommendations. If you do not take diabetes medication, you may not need to test as often as someone who does. At least two days per week, you should test in the morning before breakfast and perhaps just before or two hours after each meal. If you take diabetes medication, especially if you use an intensive insulin routine involving multiple daily injections or an insulin pump, you need to test much more frequently—usually before each meal and at bedtime. Follow these general guidelines for testing:

- Test anytime you do not feel right. Low blood glucose may be the cause of a headache, hunger, unusual fatigue, weakness, shakiness, or inability to concentrate. These are also symptoms of anxiety and normal hunger, however, so it's important to test.

- Test before and after eating foods you suspect cause your glucose level to run high or low. Then the next time you eat that food, you can adjust your insulin or the amount you eat.

- Once a week, test your glucose during the night—say, between 2 and 4 A.M.

- Test frequently when you are sick. If you are vomiting or are very ill, test at least every two hours and perform a urine ketone test at least every 24 hours (see Remedy 27).

- Test before driving a vehicle. Test every two hours during car trips.

- Test if you're unsure whether to eat. If you're dining out and dinner might be late, a test can help you decide if you should have a snack.

- Test during the peak action times of your insulin (see Remedy 37). For example, Regular insulin peaks two to four hours after injection. Therefore, if you take Regular insulin at 7 A.M., you might test your blood around 9:30 or 10 A.M.

- Test before and after you exercise. Glucose levels can continue to fall for up to 24 hours after strenuous exercise, even after an insulin injection.

TAKE MEDICINE PROPERLY.

Whether you take insulin injections or an oral agent (pill) to lower your blood glucose, it is critical that you take the right dose at the right time. Make sure you know the type and dose of your medication, when it starts to lower blood glucose, when it works hardest (peaks), and how long it is effective.

If you take an oral agent:

- Ask your diabetes educator or doctor what to do if you miss a dose. If you completely miss a dose, do not double up on your next dose.

- Know if you should take your medication on an empty stomach or with food.

- Recognize the signs of hypoglycemia (low blood glucose). See Remedy 36 for more information.

- Report any side effects, such as stomach problems or rashes, to your doctor.

If you take insulin, your diabetes educator will show you the proper technique for giving yourself an insulin injection. Each time you give yourself a shot, keep the following in mind:

- Roll NPH, Lente, or Ultralente insulin to mix it before drawing it up into the syringe.

- Always draw air into the syringe in the amount of your dose, and inject this air into the insulin bottle. Replacing the insulin you remove with air prevents the airtight bottle from developing a vacuum. If you don't perform this step, it will become more difficult to remove the insulin each time.

- If you mix insulins, always do it in the same order so you do not confuse your doses. Draw up Regular into the syringe first, then NPH.

- Check for air bubbles. If injected into your skin, an air bubble will not hurt you, but its presence probably means you're not getting the correct dose of insulin. If you see a bubble, push the insulin back into the bottle and draw it up again.

- Make sure you've measured accurately. If necessary, ask a family member or friend to double-check your dose. If you have trouble seeing the lines on the syringe, try holding it in front of something white. If this technique doesn't help, magnifiers that clamp around the syringe are available at most pharmacies.

- Pinch the skin where you wish to inject the insulin. Inject insulin straight in at a 90-degree angle.

- If you have trouble with insulin leaking at injection sites, pull the skin to one side before inserting the needle and count to 10 before pulling the needle out. Make sure you release the pinched skin before you pull the needle out. The pressure of the pinch can force insulin out the hole.

- If occasionally you find it hard to push the insulin in, pull the needle back a bit and try again. If it still does not plunge, start again with a new syringe.

- If you have frequent bruising or unusual pain at your injection sites, let your diabetes educator or doctor watch your injection technique.

WRITE IT DOWN.

Keeping records of every test, every result, every dose, every symptom, and every sign can be tedious, but it is one of the best ways for you and your doctor to assess the success of diabetes control. Excellent record keeping allows you to identify patterns of high and low blood glucose levels, the effects of certain foods, and your body's response to exercise.

Here are some guidelines to help make record keeping easier:

- Keep your record and a pen or pencil near your meter or, if possible, in the case so you are more likely to fill it in immediately. Don't rely on memory (yours or the meter's) to catch up on your record keeping.

- If you have an active day, either at work or play, make a note of this. When you look back in your record, these notes can help explain why numbers were a bit lower than usual that day.

- If you are sick, if you eat more or less than you usually do, or if your schedule was off on any given day, write this down.

- If you experience low blood glucose and treat for it, write this down.

- Write down any blood glucose results you obtain in between your usual test times, additional insulin doses, and use of any other medication—prescription or over the counter—such as antibiotics or cold remedies.

- Study your records periodically. Are the numbers where you want them to be? Do you see any patterns of control? (See also Remedy 42.)

- Always take your records with you to doctor appointments.

15 EXERCISE!

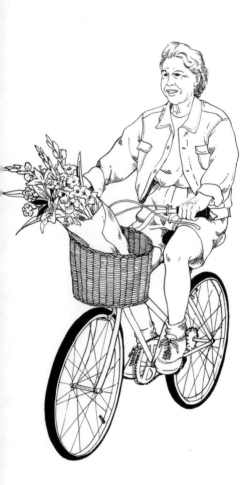

Join the many people who have discovered that exercise makes them look and feel better. Among its benefits, regular exercise lowers blood glucose and cholesterol levels; reduces your risk of high blood pressure, heart attack, and stroke; and improves bone density, your mood, and your figure. There's no doubt exercise greatly benefits people with diabetes. So find an activity or two you enjoy, and fit exercise into your diabetes management. Note: If you are overweight or older than 40 years of age, check with your doctor before you begin an exercise program.

- Set up a regular time in your schedule to exercise. To add even more incentive, get a friend or family member to exercise with you!

- Warm up before and cool down after any exercise session. Perform stretches as well as light aerobic exercises, such as marching in place, to get the blood moving into your muscles.

- Wear comfortable gear appropriate for the temperature and activity. Layer clothes so you can peel down when you begin to sweat. Make sure you wear thick or even double socks if you are prone to blisters.

- Test blood glucose levels before and after exercise. If you usually exercise for longer than 30 minutes, and your blood glucose is usually in your target range, plan to eat more before, during, and after exercise. If you take insulin, you can also consider adjusting your dose before exercise.

- Always have a simple sugar handy when you exercise in case you experience low blood glucose. Eat it if you feel unusually uncoordinated, sweaty, or light-headed. When you exercise strenuously or for a long period, take a break for some juice or a snack to keep your blood glucose levels up. A general rule of thumb: Eat 15 grams of carbohydrate for each hour of moderate activity.

- Drink plenty of water before, during, and after exercising.

- Ask your doctor or diabetes educator about exercise precautions when your insulin is peaking, when you have ketones in your urine, or when you exercise more than two hours after eating.

PLAN YOUR DIET.

16

Thoughtful meal planning has always been the cornerstone of diabetes treatment. If you have Type II diabetes, nutrition planning may be your only course of treatment. If you require a pill or insulin, you must balance your medication and exercise therapy with meal planning.

But if you thought that having diabetes meant you could never again enjoy a dish of ice cream, you may be in for a very pleasant surprise. In May 1994, the American Diabetes Association and the American Dietetic Association drafted new nutrition guidelines for the management of diabetes. The new guidelines prescribe a diet based on an individual's metabolism, lifestyle, and nutritional needs, instead of the traditional calorie-based plan. The goals of the new guidelines are to help people with diabetes achieve a reasonable weight and normal blood glucose levels, lipid levels (particularly cholesterol and triglycerides), and blood pressure.

The new nutrition guidelines may also make your life a little sweeter. They emphasize *total* carbohydrate intake—whether the carbohydrate source is sugar or starch, cake or mashed potatoes. Research has demonstrated that all carbohydrates end up as glucose; it's just a matter of time. So nutrition experts now consider all carbohydrates as one food category. You may consume some sugary foods in place of some starchy foods as long as you don't exceed your recommended total intake of carbohydrate for the day or meal.

You should work with a registered dietitian to create a meal plan tailored to your current and desirable body weight; eating and exercise patterns; blood glucose and hemoglobin A_{1C} records; and any medication you take.

Here are some tips for a successful meal plan:

- Determine your most important goal in managing diabetes and planning your diet. Do you want to lose weight? Make more nutritious food choices? Tell your registered dietitian your goals and in what areas you need the most help.

- Check your progress. Monitor blood glucose, hemoglobin A_{1C} results, lipid levels, and any weight loss.

- Keep good records. Identify areas where you're doing well and where you're having difficulty.

- Maintain a regular schedule. Consistency in timing and amount of food is important for people who require insulin. You must also learn to balance food with the actions of insulin on days when your schedule changes or when you are more or less active than usual.

- Space meals and snacks throughout the day, instead of eating only three meals.

- Lose weight if you need to. Extra body fat makes it harder for the body to produce insulin to match your intake of food. As a result, you require more insulin to balance glucose levels. Weight loss allows the insulin to work more effectively. Many people have decreased their insulin dose after weight loss.

- Use the Food Guide Pyramid shown to plan a balanced diet.

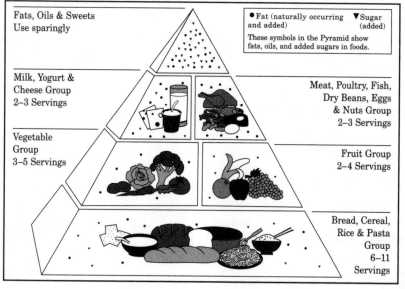

Fats, Oils & Sweets
Use sparingly

● Fat (naturally occurring and added)   ▼ Sugar (added)

These symbols in the Pyramid show fats, oils, and added sugars in foods.

Milk, Yogurt & Cheese Group
2–3 Servings

Vegetable Group
3–5 Servings

Meat, Poultry, Fish, Dry Beans, Eggs & Nuts Group
2–3 Servings

Fruit Group
2–4 Servings

Bread, Cereal, Rice & Pasta Group
6–11 Servings

The Food Guide Pyramid was designed to help people make healthier food choices. Build your diet from the bottom up. The location of food groups on the Pyramid corresponds with the number of recommended servings you should eat daily. You should try to eat the most servings from the group at the Pyramid base—bread, cereal, rice, and pasta—and the fewest from the Pyramid tip—fats, oils, and sweets.

Portion sizes are important in balancing blood glucose levels. You will learn techniques to estimate portion sizes, including these:

A closed fist is roughly a cup.

The size of your thumb is approximately 1 ounce of cheese.

A 3- to 4-ounce serving of meat or fish is about the size and thickness of a woman's palm.

BE A LABEL READER.

If you haven't noticed, food package labels are now worthwhile reading. A gift to consumers from our federal friends, the Nutrition Labeling and Education Act of 1990 requires manufacturers to put specific nutrition information on food labels. The new labels make it easy to select foods that fit into your meal plan. The labels list, for one serving, the nutrients most relevant to your health: total and saturated fats, cholesterol, sodium, carbohydrates, dietary fiber, sugars, proteins, and vitamins and minerals. Serving sizes are now standardized to help you make better-informed choices. The column % Daily Value shows how this food fits into a daily diet of 2,000 calories.

The nutrition label is not the only label you should understand. What about all those claims a food is "lite" or "fat free"? Can you believe them? Now you can. Claims on product labels must meet legal standards set by the government. Here's a dictionary of claims:

If the label says:	The product contains, per serving:
Sugar free	less than ½ gram of sugar
Nonfat or Fat free	½ gram of fat or less
Low fat	3 grams of fat or less
Reduced fat	25% less saturated fat than similar foods
Lean	less than 10 grams of fat, 4 grams of saturated fat, and 95 milligrams of cholesterol
Extra lean	less than 5 grams of fat, 2 grams of saturated fat, and 95 milligrams of cholesterol
Calorie free	less than 5 calories
Low calorie	40 calories or less
Reduced calorie	At least 25% fewer calories than similar foods
Light or Lite	⅓ fewer calories or 50% less fat

Low cholesterol	20 milligrams or less cholesterol and 2 grams or less saturated fat
Cholesterol free	Less than 2 milligrams cholesterol and 2 grams or less saturated fat
High fiber	5 grams of fiber or more

Talk to your dietitian to learn more about fitting different foods into your meal plan. Save the labels from foods you have questions about so your dietitian can help you figure out how to plug them into your meal plan.

A caution to those who use the American Diabetes Association Exchange List: The standard serving sizes listed on the product label may differ from the size listed on the exchange list. For example, a standard serving size of fruit juice is 8 ounces, but the exchange lists a fruit juice serving size as 4 ounces.

Serving Size ——

Nutrition Facts

Serving Size ½ cup (114g)
Servings per Container 4

Amount Per Serving

| Calories 90 | Calories from Fat 30 |
| | **% Daily Value*** |

Calories from Fat ——

	% Daily Value
Total Fat 3g	5%
Saturated Fat 0g	0%
Cholesterol 0mg	0%
Sodium 300mg	13%
Total Carbohydrate 13g	4%
Dietary Fiber 3g	12%
Sugars 3g	
Protein 3g	

% Daily Value panel ——

List of nutrients ——

| Vitamin A 80% | • | Vitamin C 60% |
| Calcium 4% | • | Iron 4% |

Vitamins and minerals ——

*Percent Daily Values are based on a 2,000 calorie diet. Your daily values may be higher or lower depending on your calorie needs.

	Calories:	2,000	2,500
Total Fat	Less than	65g	80g
Sat Fat	Less than	20g	25g
Cholesterol	Less than	300mg	300mg
Sodium	Less than	2,400mg	2,400mg
Total Carbohydrate		300g	375g
Fiber		25g	30g

Daily Value panel ——

Calories per gram:

Fat 9 • Carbohydrate 4 • Protein 4

MAKE EXCHANGES IN YOUR DIET.

Exactly what effect does the food you eat have on your blood glucose? In a nutshell, carbohydrates (sugars and starches) account for most of the glucose in your blood. About half the protein you eat could convert to glucose. But it's pretty tough for the body to turn fat into glucose. As you probably already figured out, most fat gets stored in the body.

Of course, when you have diabetes, it is important to try to maintain an even level of glucose in the blood, and you do so by balancing food and exercise and perhaps medication. To maintain this balance, many people with diabetes follow an exchange diet. An exchange diet allows you to eat a wide variety of foods, while keeping blood glucose levels stable.

The exchange diet divides foods into six groups: Starch/Bread, Meat, Vegetable, Fruit, Milk, and Fat. Foods in each group have similar amounts of carbohydrate, protein, and fat. When digested, each food in the group turns into an approximately equal amount of glucose. For example, one Starch/Bread exchange includes the following foods: ½ bagel, 1 slice of toast, ½ cup shredded wheat, ½ cup oatmeal, or ½ English muffin. Each of these foods contains about 15 grams of carbohydrate, 3 grams of protein, a trace of fat, and 80 calories. So if your meal plan calls for one Starch/Bread exchange for breakfast, you can choose from among these different foods.

As you can see from the example, portion sizes may differ. This is because the total weight of the foods differs; for example, the portion size is larger for puffed rice because it weighs less than Grape Nuts. Other factors also affect how much glucose each food produces, including whether the food is cooked and whether it contains fat or fiber. So the ½ bagel may cause your blood glucose to run higher than the ½ cup of oatmeal. You need to experiment and test your blood glucose level after eating certain foods. A registered dietitian or your diabetes educator can get you started on an exchange diet and provide you with exchange charts to map the way.

19 LEAN AWAY FROM FAT.

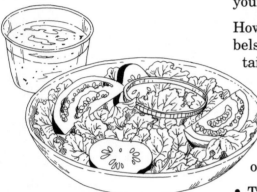

We know we should reduce the amount of fat in our diets. If we do, researchers say, we'll lose weight, prevent some types of disease, and probably feel better. But reducing fat is hard, right? Wrong! Reducing fat in your diet isn't as tough as you might think.

How do you start? First, pay attention to the type of fat you eat. Read labels; they indicate how much total fat and saturated fat a product contains. Saturated fats are implicated in raising the blood cholesterol level and clogging the arteries. You'll find saturated fats in all animal products, as well as in coconut and palm oils. These fats are solid at room temperature (think of butter and shortening). Choose heart-healthier unsaturated fats such as polyunsaturated corn, safflower, sunflower, and soybean oils and monounsaturated olive and canola oil. Here are just a few other ways you can reduce fat in your diet:

- Trim fat from meats and remove skin from poultry before eating.

- Bake, broil, poach, or steam foods instead of frying. Season foods with herbs and spices instead of butter, margarine, or a sauce.

- Ask for sauces and dressings to be served "on the side." Then dip your fork lightly in these side dishes to get the flavor.

- Make substitutions. Substitute low-fat frozen yogurt for ice cream, skim milk for low-fat or whole milk, fat-free salad dressing for regular dressing. Experiment with recipes. In baked goods, for example, you can substitute unsweetened applesauce for oil.

- Eat more vegetables, less meat. Veggies fill you up and add fiber to your diet (see Remedy 20).

- When dining out, ask how food is prepared. If the scrod is broiled in lemon butter, ask if they can broil it in orange juice instead.

One last note: Just because a label claims the food is low or nonfat, it doesn't necessarily mean the food is better for you. Some manufacturers increase the amount of protein, sodium, and/or sugar when they remove the fat—and keep all the calories.

FIT IN FIBER.

By now you've heard all the claims about the benefits of fiber. This is one area where you can believe what you hear. Including a source of fiber at every meal can have the following benefits:

• Fiber takes up space in your stomach and small intestine before it is excreted, and actually may cause you to eat less because you feel full faster.

• It adds bulk to your diet, preventing constipation and hemorrhoids.

• It triggers less of a rise in blood glucose levels than other nutrients, and the effect remains a while due to slower absorption of food.

• It may reduce the risk of colon and rectal cancers.

• It lowers cholesterol.

Fiber is actually a group of widely different plant carbohydrates. What they have in common is that the human digestive tract does not completely digest and absorb them as it does other forms of carbohydrate. Fiber is found in unrefined grains such as whole wheat, rye, corn, oats, and brown rice; dried beans and peas; and all fruits and vegetables. Most nutrition experts suggest consuming 20 to 35 grams of fiber each day. Try the following tips for boosting your fiber intake:

• When you have a choice, choose food high in fiber. Choose whole-grain breads instead of refined white, bran cereal instead of plain cornflakes, brown rice instead of white, whole wheat instead of regular pasta.

• Leave the edible skins on fresh fruits and vegetables. These skins are an excellent source of fiber.

• Eat a piece of fresh fruit rather than drinking juice. An orange has more fiber than orange juice.

• Read labels for the amount of fiber the food contains. (See Remedy 17.)

• Drink plenty of water. If fiber does not absorb enough water, it can slow rather than speed up elimination.

SET ASIDE THE SALT SHAKER.

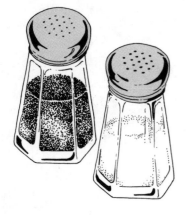

Even if you wanted to, you probably couldn't eliminate sodium completely from your diet. Sodium is in just about everything—from water to vegetables—and it is important to your health. But there are good reasons to watch your sodium intake.

Sodium controls fluid balance in the body. Too much sodium causes bloating, swelling, and excess water weight. In people who are sensitive to sodium's effects, it has been linked to elevated blood pressure (hypertension). Hypertension increases your risk of heart attack, stroke, kidney failure, and buildup of plaque in the arteries (atherosclerosis). These complications are even more likely to occur in people with diabetes. Because no test can tell you if you're "salt sensitive," it makes sense to be careful about salt intake. People with diabetes should not exceed more than 2,400 milligrams of sodium per day. Here are a few ideas to reduce your salt intake:

- Keep the salt shaker off the table.

- Don't salt foods when cooking—even when a recipe calls for added salt.

- Buy reduced-sodium canned soups and vegetables. (Frozen vegetables are usually sodium-free and cheaper, too.)

- Limit your intake of certain condiments, such as ketchup, mustard, and soy, barbecue, and Worcestershire sauces.

- Learn to spice up your foods with lemon, herbs, and spices instead of salt.

- Read food labels carefully for sodium content. A good rule of thumb is the food should not contain more than 1 to 2 milligrams of sodium per calorie.

SUPPLEMENT IF YOU MUST.

Should you take a vitamin or mineral supplement? Most registered dietitians advocate getting the bulk of your nutrients from food sources. To achieve a healthy diet, you should consume at least six servings from the grain group daily and five or more servings from the fruits and vegetables group. Although it is too early to recommend supplementation for everyone with diabetes, there is accumulating scientific evidence that certain supplements may be beneficial for those with specific needs or complications. Those who are at higher risk for deficiency include:

- Those on very low-calorie diets (1,200 calories or less per day)

- Pregnant and breast-feeding women, vegetarians, and the elderly

- Those taking a medication known to cause a vitamin or mineral deficiency

- Those with complications of diabetes: kidney failure, cardiovascular disease, hypertension, neuropathy, persistent hyperglycemia (high blood glucose) accompanied by glycosuria (sugar in the urine)

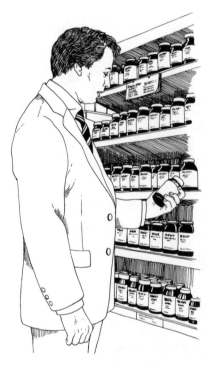

Many health experts believe that women should take calcium supplements throughout adolescence and adulthood to prevent osteoporosis. Low doses of vitamin B_6 (25 milligrams twice a day) have been shown to relieve symptoms of peripheral neuropathy (nerve damage) in some people with diabetes. Magnesium supplementation may be required particularly in Type II diabetes, since many people with this condition follow lower calorie diets and may be eating fewer meat and dairy products. You may have heard otherwise, but chromium supplementation does not improve diabetes control unless you already have a deficiency. However, chromium deficiency is rare. Persons on low-fat diets may require vitamin E in amounts from 400 to 800 milligrams per day. Vitamin E has been shown to reduce the amount of heart-damaging cholesterol. Ask your doctor and registered dietitian to evaluate your diet and overall diabetes status. They may recommend supplements for you based on your circumstances.

KNOW HOW ALCOHOL FITS IN.

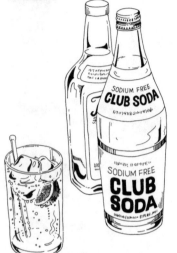

In most cases, you can fit one or two alcoholic drinks into your meal plan with little effect on blood glucose levels. But do recognize that alcohol's effects may be cause for concern.

Alcohol blocks the liver from releasing glucose during periods of fasting (overnight or between meals), which can lead to hypoglycemia: This effect can last from 8 to 12 hours after drinking, particularly among insulin users. High blood pressure is associated with drinking three or more drinks per day, and people with diabetes already have a high risk of developing high blood pressure. The peripheral nerves (nerves that go to the hands and feet) can be very sensitive to excessive levels of alcohol in the blood. This suggests that nerve damage could progress more quickly with regular alcohol use. Follow this advice when you drink alcohol:

- Choose "lite" beers or dry white wine. Mix drinks with diet soda, club soda, or water to dilute them. Sweet wines, liqueurs, fruit drinks, or drinks made with regular soda usually raise blood glucose levels. Make your own drink when possible, so you know exactly what's in it!

- Don't drink on an empty stomach. Drink with a meal or after eating.

- Drink slowly. Limit yourself to two drinks; make them last.

- Count alcohol calories. Count 1 ounce of alcohol as 2 fat exchanges. Check labels for carbohydrate content. If you adjust your insulin to your diet, you probably will need less insulin when you drink alcohol.

- Test your blood glucose before, during, and after drinking. If you are intoxicated, you may not recognize signs of hypoglycemia.

- Make sure you're with someone who knows you have diabetes and knows the signs of and treatment for hypoglycemia.

Finally, use of alcohol with some diabetes medications can cause flushing of the face and neck, mild sweating, and, in some cases, headache, nausea, palpitations, and breathlessness. If you experience this problem, ask your doctor if you can switch medications.

HINT

Here are calories of common alcoholic beverages.

Beer, light, 12 fl oz 95

Beer, regular, 12 fl oz . .150

Gin, rum, vodka, whiskey, tequila, 80-proof, 1½ fl oz 97

Gin, rum, vodka, whiskey, tequila, 90-proof, 1½ fl oz . . .110

Wine, red, 3½ fl oz 74

Wine, white, 3½ fl oz . . .70

PLAN FOR PARTIES.

Participating in special events with friends and family and taking care of diabetes need not be at odds with each other! But it can seem a bit tricky. If you're going out for brunch, do you call it breakfast or lunch? When should you take insulin? How do you manage a 3 P.M. dinner? Should you eat again at 6 P.M.?

If you control diabetes with diet or pills alone, an occasional deviation from your schedule is generally not critical. If you take insulin, you can plan ahead to fit in the schedule changes. If you are the kind of person who is always ready for a spontaneous party, you should consider a multiple daily injection routine or insulin pump to give your schedule more flexibility (see Remedy 39).

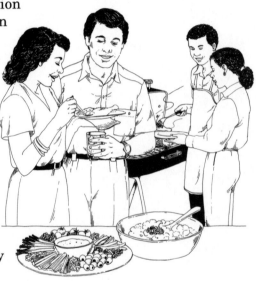

If you take insulin, and you've kept careful records, you'll be able to tell when your insulin works hardest and when it does not work well. Does the time of the change you wish to make fall within a pattern of high glucose levels? If so, it's OK to delay your meal, or you can subtract one to two servings of your usual carbohydrate servings (fruit, milk, and/or starches) from the meal. Generally, one serving raises blood glucose about 50 points, so subtract accordingly. If you take insulin, another alternative is to take extra insulin before the meal. Again, generally, 1 unit of Regular insulin decreases blood glucose by about 50 points (it also covers about 15 grams of carbohydrate).

If the change falls during a low pattern, you could decrease the amount of Regular insulin you take, using the same rule of thumb described above, or simply plan to eat more. You can also change the timing of the insulin and the amount, but you must plan ahead for it. Contact your diabetes educator to help you work out a plan.

Also consider these tips for planning ahead:

- If you're dining with friends, ask your hosts these questions: What foods will they serve? What time? Will they serve snacks before dinner? If the event is a cocktail party, will food be available? (Consider if any appetizers will be the type you can make a meal out of.) Will they serve dessert at the time of the meal or later in the evening? Remember, if your friends know you have diabetes, these questions will not be awkward for you or them. Decide if the foods available are appropriate for your needs or if you need to supplement them or adjust your insulin. If mealtime is uncertain, you may not want to take insulin until you are sure food is available. Always carry glucose tablets, or ask for crackers, juice, or soda if a meal is delayed.

- Offer to bring a dish: a vegetable snack tray or a salad if the planned menu consists of tempting high fat foods, or a dessert that is healthy and appropriate for you. Offer to bring diet drinks, or place a six-pack in your car in case none is available.

- Follow the same suggestions for restaurant dining. Call ahead to ask what selections are on the menu. If dinner is delayed, ask the waiter for bread or crackers to tide you over. (Test blood glucose if you can: If it is normal or high, you can wait for dinner without a problem.) Again, hold off taking your insulin until the food is served.

- Try to stay within 1 to 1½ hours of your usual schedule. If this is not possible, talk to your doctor about taking intermediate-acting insulin at the usual time and moving the Regular insulin to 30 minutes before you eat. You may need to adjust your dose if you do this.

- Decide ahead of time how you will handle special foods. Will you eat dessert and take extra insulin to compensate, or will you skip some other part of the meal and take your usual dose? A registered dietitian can help you figure any exchanges (see Remedy 18).

- Plan for any alcoholic beverages (see Remedy 23).

- Experiment! Try one method to maintain blood glucose levels this time and another method the next time a special circumstance arises. Keep good records so you can see what worked and plan for the next time.

Recognize that control doesn't always work perfectly. You may need to settle for less-than-optimal control on days your schedule is off. Do the best you can, but don't give up participating in activities you enjoy. Have a good time!

PAMPER YOUR FEET.

Whether you have Type I or Type II diabetes, it is important to take good care of your feet. The best way to do this is with good glucose control. Like other complications of diabetes, foot problems develop from nerve and blood vessel damage that occurs when blood glucose levels are persistently high for a number of years. The excess glucose coats the nerve cells and narrows the small blood vessels to the feet, accelerating the process that causes atherosclerosis (the buildup of fatty deposits on the inner lining of the blood vessels). Other factors such as a family history of heart disease and unhealthy lifestyle choices (smoking, high-fat diet, lack of exercise) also increase your risk of nerve and blood vessel damage.

High blood glucose levels also increase your risk of infection. Bacteria love to grow on sugar in tissues, and white cells can't battle the infection effectively when they're sticky with sugar. If not treated early, infections or ulcers of the feet can develop into serious conditions.

Nerve damage can develop slowly; you may not even be aware of a problem. Warnings of nerve damage include pain, burning, tingling or a "pins and needles" feeling, or numbness.

Follow these tips to prevent foot problems:

- Get in the habit of examining your feet after your shower or bath. Notify your doctor of any redness, blisters, corns, scrapes, cracks, or swelling. Make sure your doctor examines your feet at every checkup.

- Wash your feet every day with a mild soap and warm water. Dry your feet thoroughly, including between the toes.

- Lower the temperature of your water tank to 120 degrees Fahrenheit. Your bath water should be about 90 degrees. Test water temperature with your elbow before putting your feet into the bath tub. Your feet may not be as sensitive to temperature, and you can burn yourself.

- Avoid soaking your feet; this dries out the skin, resulting in cracks that could become infected. Avoid use of strong chemicals such as Epsom salts or iodine in your bath water.

WARNING

Never cut your corns or callouses.

Never treat corns and callouses yourself with over-the-counter remedies.

Never treat an ingrown toenail yourself. See a doctor for treatment.

- Moisturize your feet with lotion. Try products that contain lanolin. Bag balm and udder cream, available at hardware, seed and feed, and many drugstores, are inexpensive medicated lanolin spreads.

- Keep your toenails trimmed. If you're not sure how to do this properly, consult your doctor. (Trimming nails is easiest immediately after a shower or bath.) If you can't see well or have trouble reaching your feet, see your doctor or a podiatrist (foot doctor).

- Always wear socks or stockings to prevent friction or rubbing of shoes against bare skin. Wear cotton socks instead of nylon when possible. Cotton allows your feet to "breathe," keeping your feet dry and cool. Avoid wearing mended socks. The darned areas can cause blisters.

- Make sure your shoes are comfortable and the right size. When purchasing new shoes, match the shape of the shoe to your foot. Trace an outline of your bare foot while standing, and use this tracing to match against new shoes. If new shoes are stiff or they rub, have them stretched or softened. Break in new shoes gradually.

- Check your shoes and socks before you put them on. Put your hand inside them to make sure no objects have found their way inside. People with nerve disease can injure their feet because they may not feel objects inside their shoes.

- Protect your feet from the cold. Wear warm socks or fleece-lined boots in cold temperatures. Wear socks at night. But do not use heating pads or hot water bottles to keep your feet warm; they can cause burns.

- Avoid wearing tight socks or garters. Support hosiery is fine because it prevents blood from pooling in the feet and legs. Remove hosiery daily for foot washing and inspection, and wear clean hose each day.

- Wear shoes whenever possible, even at home. Going barefoot increases your risk of foot injury.

- If you have nerve or circulatory problems in your feet, consider purchasing therapeutic shoes. These shoes support the pressure points and reduce stress on your feet when you walk. Therapeutic shoes are now reimbursed by Medicare if you have a doctor's prescription.

SEE YOUR EYE DOCTOR.

Uncontrolled diabetes can lead to serious eye disease (retinopathy) and loss of vision. That's the bad news. The good news is that by keeping blood glucose levels near normal, you can reduce your risk of eye disease up to 70 percent!

The leading cause of new cases of adult blindness in the United States (some 39,000 every year) is diabetic retinopathy. Your risk of retinopathy is related to how long you've had diabetes, your level of glucose control, and whether you have high blood pressure (hypertension). Hypertension increases pressure on blood vessels, while persistent high blood glucose (hyperglycemia) causes narrowing of them.

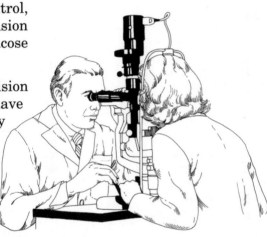

You may notice that when your blood glucose levels are high, your vision is blurry. Signs may look blurred at a distance or you may find you have more difficulty reading. This is not a sign of eye disease; it is caused by the lens in your eye changing shape with glucose and water shifts in your body. It usually clears up when blood glucose levels return to normal. People also notice blurred vision for a short time (a few days to a few weeks) after they begin taking insulin. If blurred vision does not clear up, consult an ophthalmologist (eye doctor).

If your sight is poor, ask your educator or eye doctor to recommend glasses or other devices to assist you. Magnifiers can help you measure insulin accurately. Glucose meters for the visually impaired are available.

But you can prevent eye problems. Follow this advice:

- See your ophthalmologist at least once a year, particularly if you have had Type I diabetes for five or more years.

- If you notice flashing lights, dark spots, or floaters that block your vision, call your eye doctor immediately.

- If you wear contact lenses, it is especially important to stick to your doctor's recommendations regarding wear, cleansing, and use of saline drops. If your eyes become too dry, your cornea may be more susceptible to injury and, once injured, may not heal well.

ADJUST FOR SICK DAYS

SICK-DAY FOOD IDEAS

These foods and beverages contain 15 grams of carbohydrate.

4 oz of regular soda

4 oz of juice (apple, orange, grape)

8 oz of Gatorade

1 Popsicle

6 LifeSaver candies

½ cup of sherbet

½ cup of gelatin (not sugarfree)

1 slice of toast or bread

3 graham crackers

6 soda crackers

6 vanilla wafers

1 oz of pretzels

½ cup of cooked cereal

½ cup of rice

fruit (small apple, pear, ½ banana, or ½ cup of fruit cocktail)

Everyone gets sick sometimes. But when you cannot eat or exercise as usual, the change in your routine combined with the stress of the illness can significantly impact diabetes control.

When you're ill, your body produces stress hormones that cause blood glucose levels to go up and may produce ketones. However, glucose levels may drop if you have nausea, vomiting, diarrhea, or poor appetite. It is extremely important to test blood glucose levels and your urine for ketones frequently during illness.

Follow this advice during an illness:

- Always take your insulin or medication. Don't make the mistake of thinking that because you're vomiting and you have no food in your stomach, you don't need to take insulin. You may need to adjust the dose, however. When vomiting is a symptom, you might need extra insulin due to the stress of the illness itself.

- Test your blood glucose every two hours when you experience vomiting or diarrhea. Test at least four times a day if you have a cold or fever.

- Test urine for ketones frequently. If the amount of ketones is small, drink fluids and continue to monitor them. If ketones persist or if levels are moderate or large, call your doctor.

- Drink plenty of fluids. Try to take in about 8 ounces of fluid per hour. If you are vomiting, sip flat regular soda. If blood glucose levels are high, drink sugar-free beverages. If glucose levels run low, drink regular soda or fruit juice.

- Consult your doctor before taking over-the-counter cold and flu medications. Some medications can affect glucose levels or produce side effects you may confuse with hypoglycemia.

- Eat small meals or snacks frequently. Try to eat and drink foods that contain enough carbohydrate to replace what you normally eat in your meal plan but are more easily digested.

Keep good records of your blood and urine tests, food, beverages, and symptoms. And keep in touch with your health care team. Call your doctor or diabetes educator if:

- you have been vomiting or have diarrhea for more than 24 hours

- you cannot eat or drink

- your blood glucose is greater than 240 milligrams/deciliter (mg/dL) or less than 80 mg/dL for more than 48 hours

- you have a temperature of 101 degrees or greater for two or more days

- you have ketones in your urine

- you have signs of ketoacidosis (see Remedy 38)

- you have chest pain

- you don't know what to do to manage your illness and diabetes

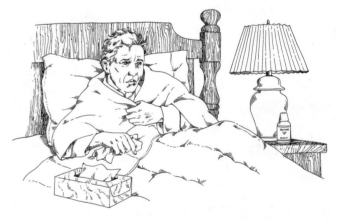

Be prepared to provide your doctor or educator with the following information:

- how long you have been ill and your symptoms (take your temperature before you call)

- blood glucose and urine ketone results for at least the past 24 hours up to the present

- the amount of insulin you've taken

- the last time you ate or drank, what, and how much

- how you have been treating your illness (over-the-counter medications, fluids, and so on)

- the telephone number of your pharmacy

- if you are allergic to any medications

DON'T GIVE YOUR MOUTH THE BRUSH-OFF.

High blood glucose levels can make people with diabetes more prone to diseases of the teeth and gums. That's because, most often, disease results from bacterial infection in the gums. Bacteria love dark, moist places such as your mouth, and the higher levels of glucose in your saliva actually nourish them. As Remedy 25 described, infection-fighting white cells sticky with sugar can't fight bacteria effectively; glucose acts as kryptonite to the white-cell Supermen. The stress of fighting an infection can cause glucose levels to continue to rise. To sum it up: Dark, moist places + high glucose content = Bacteria that thrive and multiply!

Properly caring for teeth and gums and keeping blood glucose levels in control are the best ways to help your body fight infection and prevent dental disease. Dental infections, or abscesses, are common with more serious dental disease and can cause blood glucose levels to go up. If you have an infection, you may need to adjust your medication.

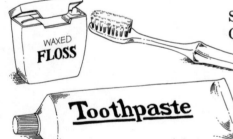

Some types of dental disease are common in people with diabetes. Gingivitis is a reversible condition affecting the gums. Caused by a buildup of bacteria and plaque on the teeth, gingivitis results in sore, swollen, red gums that may bleed easily when you floss or brush. (Plaque is the thin, whitish film that coats the teeth and tongue. Plaque uses glucose to create an acid strong enough to dissolve the tooth's enamel.) Periodontitis, the more advanced stage of gum disease, follows untreated gingivitis. The gums pull away or shrink from your teeth, leaving pockets where bacteria breed. Periodontitis can erode the bone that supports the teeth.

Here are tips to keep your mouth healthy:

• Brush your teeth at least twice a day. After every meal or snack is better, especially if you've eaten a sweet, sticky food that will stick to your teeth. And make sure you brush before you go to bed.

- Floss your teeth every day. Flossing helps prevent plaque from forming between the teeth—where your brush can't reach.

- Use a soft toothbrush and a toothpaste with fluoride. Ask your dentist to recommend an antiseptic mouthwash that can kill the bacteria that cause plaque.

- When you can't brush your teeth, chew sugar-free gum after meals to help dislodge food particles between teeth.

- See your dentist twice a year for cleaning. Make sure he or she knows you have diabetes. Your dentist can develop a plan of care for your special needs.

- If you notice swelling, redness, bleeding or sore gums, loose teeth, or a bad taste in your mouth, see your dentist. Don't wait for a full-blown toothache; call as soon as you feel the first twinges of pain. Sometimes the right treatment early in the game can prevent more serious problems later on. Incidentally, do not put an ice pack on a dental infection. Even though it might feel good, you are shutting down blood flow to the area. Your body needs a good blood flow to fight infection.

- See your dentist regularly if you wear dentures. Dentures should be re-lined from time to time to prevent sore spots and ulcers from developing.

- Give your dentist the name and phone number of your doctor, and ask that your doctor be notified of any problems.

- Ask your dentist to consult your doctor before any dental surgery. You may need to make major adjustments in your medication depending on when the surgery takes place, the seriousness of the surgery, the type of anesthesia, and how well you will be able to eat afterward.

- If you must undergo a major dental procedure, prepare for any inability to chew. You may need to purchase some special foods for your recovery period. Look for easy-to-swallow sources of carbohydrate such as soup, shakes, ice cream, ice milk, sherbet, sorbet, or hot cereals.

- Try to arrange your dental appointments so they don't interfere with your meal schedule. Don't skip a meal or your medication before your appointment.

TOSS THE TOBACCO.

You've heard all the warnings about the use of tobacco products. But have you heeded them?

Smoking can lead to high blood pressure, heart disease, and lung disease. It can cause allergies, sinusitis, and respiratory illness. You already know that people with diabetes have an increased risk of hypertension and vascular disease. When you have diabetes and you use tobacco products, the negative effects of each are compounded, which means the risks increase significantly. Your chances of developing blood vessel, heart, kidney, and eye complications grow.

Need help to quit? Try these tips:

• Make a list of all the reasons you want to quit, and post it in a place you will see it frequently.

• Rid your home, car, workplace, purse, and pockets of cigarettes, ashtrays, matches, lighters, and anything else that would remind you to smoke. Avoid activities you associate with smoking. If you always have a cigarette with a cup of coffee, drink less coffee. If you smoke in the car to and from work, carpool with a nonsmoking friend or take public transportation for a while.

• Ask your doctor about a nicotine patch to help you with withdrawal symptoms. The patch, worn on the skin, can help you feel more comfortable while you cut back.

• Tell family and friends you're quitting so they can support you.

• Don't forget to reward yourself for a job well done! A night at the movies, dinner out, a new item of clothing—paid for with the money you saved from not buying cigarettes—can keep you motivated. For a larger reward, consider joining a health club or taking dancing lessons.

The signs of nicotine withdrawal—hunger, fatigue, drowsiness, headache, irritability, anxiety, depression—can also be signs of low blood glucose. Be sure to test your blood glucose if you experience these symptoms.

SAY NO TO DRUGS.

This remedy is very simple: Drugs impede diabetes care.

First there's the obvious problem that applies to everyone, not just people with diabetes: Using marijuana, cocaine, heroin, inhalants, amphetamines, or other drugs can lead to physical and psychological addiction. But we're not only talking about illegal drugs here. The misuse of alcohol, prescription medication, and over-the-counter drugs can be just as dangerous.

Drugs may cause you to feel you have escaped from problems or worries—but when the drug wears off, the problems are still there. Drugs can rob you of your good judgment, your ability to focus or concentrate, your desire to care about yourself and others. When it comes to diabetes, you may not be able to focus on your care or care whether you focus.

The effects of drugs on blood glucose vary. Some drugs suppress appetite, which may result in low blood glucose levels. To compound the problem, the high and low feelings you get from drugs can mask the signs of hypoglycemia (low blood glucose) or hyperglycemia (high blood glucose). You may not recognize the symptoms and, therefore, not treat the condition.

Other drugs such as marijuana may stimulate appetite. With these drugs, you may find yourself snacking all day, overeating at a meal, or, in the worst case scenario, not remembering what or if you ate, and you will end up dealing with high blood glucose levels.

If you use drugs regularly—even if you believe you are not addicted and can stop at any time—get help. Talk to a doctor, a counselor, or a clergymember or seek out a self-help group or treatment program.

31

PRACTICE LETTING GO.

It's the rare person, indeed, who does not experience stress. The rest of us are familiar with its impact. In the short-term, stress causes frowns and fatigue; you may not be able to think clearly, sleep well, or remember well. Stress can impair the body's ability to fight illness. In the long-term it can lead to depression, nervous disorders, heart disease, and other serious conditions. Stress can really mess up your diabetes control, too.

When you have diabetes, the body produces stress hormones such as adrenaline that cause blood glucose levels to run high. Students with diabetes, for example, may notice their blood glucose levels run high during final exam week, or you may find your glucose is high the day you make a major presentation at work. In general, the small daily upsets don't make much difference in blood glucose levels, but chronic stress does. It robs you of the energy you need to take good care of yourself. In some people with diabetes, the release of adrenaline and the resulting quickened metabolism may result in hypoglycemia (this is more likely to happen with a one-time stressful event as opposed to chronic stress). Blood glucose monitoring can help you identify the effects of different stress on your glucose levels.

We must all face some stress, but we can learn to better manage stressful times and maybe even eliminate some of the stress in our lives. Start with a bit of detective work. Think about what situations cause you stress, and write them down. Next, figure out what activities lift your spirits, and write those down. Clearly you want to reduce the number of entries in the first list and promote the activities in the second.

- Schedule at least one activity from your positive list each day. If you find exercise a tension-breaker, go for a walk or jog. Or maybe you prefer a leisurely bath, a nap, a massage, listening to music, or reading. Make time for these!

- Develop a network of support. People who have the most success with diabetes care have a strong social network. Call on your friends for help and support when times are rough.

- Confront your problems head on. Sometimes the more directly you address a stressful situation, the sooner you can get it behind you.

- Don't overextend yourself. Learn to say "No."

- Set specific and achievable goals, and develop tactics to allow you to attain them. For example, if dinnertime causes stress, perhaps another family member could prepare at least one meal each week or you could prepare meals ahead of time and freeze them.

- Learn relaxation techniques. Close your eyes and imagine yourself in a beautiful, relaxing place—at the beach, in the mountains, looking at a sunset. Practice relaxing all of your muscles starting with your toes and working up to your forehead. Or take time when you are tense or hurried to perform deep breathing exercises. Devote some time each day to meditation and reflection.

- Share some of the responsibilities that cause stress. Delegate some activities to the kids or your partner. Adjust your budget so you can hire someone occasionally to do some of the tasks you usually do yourself— cutting the grass or cleaning the house. Remember, your time is valuable, too.

- Try something new. Developing new interests helps you widen your circle of friends and relieves your stress.

- Think positively. Concentrate on what is going well for you and what you do well.

- Maintain your sense of humor. Don't take yourself too seriously! Even living with diabetes can have its humorous moments.

GET HELP WHEN YOU NEED IT.

Juggling all of life's normal demands is hard enough. Add diabetes control to the mix and you face a tremendous challenge keeping all of the balls in the air all of the time. Sometimes you'll drop one, two, or even all of them! Wouldn't it help if someone else could carry a ball or two for a while? The point is, everybody needs help sometimes. When you can't manage life's demands as well as you usually do, you might feel blue or even depressed.

Depression is fairly common in people with a chronic illness such as diabetes. A classic definition of depression is "anger turned inward." Whether people feel angry that they have diabetes, at restrictions imposed by a diabetes regimen, at lack of control over their future well-being, or at lack of support from others, they can be vulnerable to depression. Depression can affect appetite, work performance, ability to focus, and interactions with others. It can affect diabetes control as well.

Recognize the symptoms of depression. And don't be afraid to ask for the help you need to treat it. Seek counseling if you are experiencing:

- a change in sleep habits (sleeping too much or too little, waking frequently)

- a change in weight or appetite (lack of appetite or binge eating)

- inability to concentrate

- fatigue

- lack of self-esteem

- loss of motivation

- thoughts of suicide

See a counselor if you are struggling to cope, even if you do not have any of these signs of depression. Talking to an objective person can help you through the rough spots. Regular counseling and perhaps medication can help you get all the balls in the air again! Your doctor or diabetes educator can provide you with referrals for help.

IDENTIFY YOURSELF.

33

In an emergency it is critical that emergency personnel know you have diabetes. Various forms of medical identification (ID) are available: wallet cards, neck chains, bracelets, or ID tags to place on your watch. Some IDs have an 800 number that anyone can call day or night to obtain computer access to diabetes treatment information. Other IDs simply display the word "Diabetes" or "Diabetic."

- Ask your diabetes educator to provide you with descriptions or show you samples of various types of IDs.

- Choose the ID you're willing to keep on your person at all times. If you decide on a wearable ID, don't buy a silver neck chain if you would be more likely to wear a gold bracelet. Consider any additional cost of a preferable style as an important investment in your health and safety.

- Do not put a neck chain on a young child; the child could choke if the chain catches on something. Plastic tags that pin to a child's undershirt are available, or consider an ankle chain.

- Consider taping a wallet medical ID to the back of your driver's license or identification card.

SAFEGUARD YOUR SEX LIFE.

"Oh no, not this part of my life, too." If that was the first thought that popped into your head when you read this title, don't panic. As with other aspects of living with diabetes, some extra care and control can help you preserve your sex life.

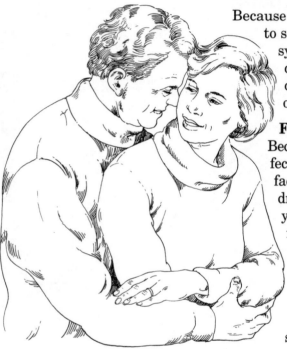

Because diabetes is a hormonal disease, it affects the systems important to sexual function: the vascular system (blood vessels), the nervous system, and the psychic (mental) system. Diabetes can alter sexual drive and performance, especially in men. It is well known that diabetes can cause impotence in men, but the effect of diabetes on female sexuality is not well understood.

For Men
Because diabetes involves the nervous and vascular systems, it can affect a man's ability to achieve or maintain an erection. Psychological factors generally play a role in impotence as well. Use of alcohol or drugs, stress, and depression can also contribute to the problem. If you are experiencing problems with impotence, your doctor may refer you to a specialist for further evaluation. You can take steps to prevent or treat diabetes-related impotence.

- Improve your blood glucose control.

- Get physically fit. Shed a few pounds. Start a strength-training program. An improved self-image can play an important role in sexual function.

- Seek counseling if you have signs of depression (see Remedy 32) or if you are having problems in your relationship with your sexual partner.

- Don't suffer in silence. Let your doctor know about any concerns you have regarding sexual performance. The problems people with diabetes face are common, and most are treatable.

For Women
Diabetes does not generally affect ovulation or fertility. But poorly controlled diabetes can result in irregular menstrual periods. Many women

also report that blood glucose levels run high a few days before the onset of their period. This might be due to hormonal fluctuations or because some women may eat more on those days.

Nerve damage that can result from prolonged periods of uncontrolled diabetes may affect sexual response in women. Hyperglycemia (high blood glucose) may lead to dehydration and decreased vaginal lubrication, which can lead to painful intercourse.

Because bacteria and yeast thrive in an environment high in sugar, women with uncontrolled diabetes are prone to vaginal infections. Yeast infections are very common; symptoms include a white or yellow cottage-cheese-like discharge, itching, burning, and, occasionally, pain. Over-the-counter treatments for yeast infections are available. Check with your doctor before using one of these products for the first time to make sure the condition is a yeast infection. (Your partner may require treatment, too.) If you have an infection, use a condom during intercourse. Otherwise you can continue to pass the infection back and forth to each other. Follow this advice to help prevent vaginal infections:

- Improve your blood glucose control.

- Use a vaginal lubricant if you are experiencing dryness or pain during intercourse. (Check with your doctor to make sure there is no other problem.)

- Wear cotton underwear, and avoid tight-fitting garments and nylon clothing that cannot "breathe." Change out of bathing suits, spandex, or exercise wear quickly to reduce your risk of a yeast infection.

- Bathe daily and always wipe front to back after voiding or bowel movements.

- See your doctor if you experience any discharge, itching, redness, or unusual odors.

- Consider use of contraceptives if blood glucose levels have not been running in your target range. Pregnancy during periods of poor control can cause birth defects and illness for the baby and complications of pregnancy for the mother (see Remedy 35).

MAINTAIN TIGHT CONTROL FOR PREGNANCY.

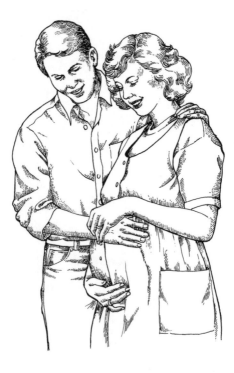

Your doctor has confirmed the news. You're pregnant! Of course, you want to do all you can for your baby. Start by giving your newborn the gift of good health.

It's true that women with diabetes have an increased risk of giving birth to babies with birth defects and illness. This risk seems to be directly related to the degree of blood glucose control, especially during the early months of pregnancy. But with good control of blood glucose levels before and throughout pregnancy, a woman with diabetes can have a healthy pregnancy and a healthy baby.

Maintaining excellent control during your pregnancy can be tricky: Your hormones rage, your weight increases, and your appetite changes. Perhaps more than at any other time, you need to work closely with your health care team to get the support you need to ensure a successful pregnancy.

Before You Become Pregnant
When you are thinking about conceiving, talk with your doctor and diabetes educator about risks to you from pregnancy. If you have long-standing diabetes, you may be at greater risk of developing or worsening certain conditions such as eye disease.

Once you decide to become pregnant, you should determine the roles and degrees of participation of different specialists in your care. Will your doctor oversee your pregnancy and delivery or will he or she refer you to an obstetrician with experience caring for women with diabetes? You will also need to select a doctor for your baby. Again, your doctor may wish to refer you to a pediatrician or neonatologist (a doctor who specializes in newborn care) with expertise in treating infants of women with diabetes. Meet these doctors ahead of time to discuss your and your baby's care.

Do your best to care for yourself! Get your blood glucose near normal and maintain the tightest control possible for several months before conceiving. This may require a lot of blood glucose testing, intensive insulin therapy, and strict adherence to a meal plan. But think of what you have to look forward to—a healthy, beautiful baby!

You should also use human insulin during this time. Animal insulin can cause antibodies to form that could harm the fetus. If you use an oral agent (pill), it should be discontinued.

During Pregnancy

Glucose testing, diligent record keeping, and close contact with your health care team are vital. Because most of the changes in metabolism and insulin will occur in the latter half of pregnancy, it's likely you'll need to increase the number of injections you administer as well as the total amount of insulin you take each day. It's not unusual to require three times more insulin during pregnancy to maintain glucose control. Also, because lower levels of blood glucose are normal for women during the latter half of pregnancy, you'll need to alter your target goals. Be sure to talk to your registered dietitian regularly throughout the pregnancy as well. You'll need to change your meal plan as your pregnancy progresses.

Follow this general advice as well:

- You should gain about one pound of weight a week during the last half of pregnancy, unless you are overweight. In that case, you should gain about one-half pound a week.

- Avoid alcohol, smoking, and all prescription and over-the-counter medications (unless prescribed by your doctor). Limit or avoid caffeine. Artificial sweeteners, including saccharin, aspartame (NutraSweet), and acesulfame K (Sweet One), are considered safe to use during pregnancy in moderate amounts.

- If you experience morning sickness, keep crackers by your bed and eat a few before you get out of bed. Eat small, frequent meals to avoid nausea.

- Watch for ketones. Periods of fasting during pregnancy are not good for you or the fetus, and ketones may have adverse effects on the baby.

- Undergo hemoglobin A_{1C} testing monthly (see Remedy 43).

- Mobilize your family and friends to help you. Allow people to help you so you can get the rest you need and stay on top of your diabetes care.

36

LOOK OUT FOR LOWS.

One of the problems with the treatment of diabetes with medication—either pills or insulin—is that hypoglycemia (low blood glucose) can occur. Hypoglycemia can occur when too much medication is in the body; you don't eat enough or a meal is delayed; or your muscles use the glucose faster than usual, such as when you exercise. Signs and symptoms of hypoglycemia, in the order they might occur, follow:

Mild	Advanced
hunger	confusion
trembling/nervousness	combativeness
sweating	disorientation
rapid pulse	unresponsiveness
pallor	seizures
headache	unconsciousness
fatigue or drowsiness	

How you treat hypoglycemia depends on: the type of diabetes you have, your size, your symptoms, the actual blood glucose level, and the recommendations of your physician or diabetes educator. There are, however, some general guidelines for treating hypoglycemia.

The first line of treatment is to eat or drink something sweet that will be absorbed into your bloodstream quickly. In a pinch, anything sweet will do, such as raisins, honey, syrup, candy, or icing. However, it is much better to take in a standard amount of glucose rather than devour everything in sight. Anxiously overeating when blood glucose levels are low may drive them too high later. The recommended amount to eat or drink when you experience hypoglycemia is 15 grams of carbohydrate, preferably in the form of 3 glucose tablets, 5 to 6 sugar cubes, or 4 to 6 ounces of fruit juice or regular soda. The amount you need may vary based on your weight and activity level and even from one episode to the next. How quickly the blood glucose level rises depends on the last time you ate, whether you exercised and the intensity of your work-out, how hard your medication is working, and whether you ate a liquid or solid food to counteract the low blood glucose (liquids absorb faster than solids).

HYPOGLYCEMIA TREATMENT

These products are recommended treatments for hypoglycemia.

3 B-D Glucose Tablets

4 CanAm's Dex 4 Tablets

1 Monogel tube (10 g carbohydrate)

5 DextroEnergy Tablets

3 Glutose Tablets

1 Glutose Gel tube (10 g carbohydrate)

1 Insta-Glucose tube (24 g carbohydrate)

3 pieces hard candy

5 LifeSavers

4 to 6 ounces fruit juice or regular soda

1 piece of fruit

4 teaspoons sugar

1 tablespoon honey or jelly

Plan how you will treat hypoglycemia before it occurs:

- Carry some form of sugar with you at all times. (See the sidebar for suggestions.) Ask friends and family to carry something sweet, too.

- Don't use chocolate candy to treat low blood glucose. Its high fat content slows the absorption of sugar, so it does not work quickly enough.

- Wait about 15 minutes before consuming more sugar, especially if you have recently eaten a meal or snack.

- Follow the glucose tablets or juice with a combination of protein and carbohydrate, such as crackers with cheese, half a sandwich, or a small bowl of cereal with milk. The carbohydrate acts to get the glucose up; the protein maintains the increased level.

- If hypoglycemia occurs around meal or snack time, go ahead and eat your meal or snack. It may help to eat your fruit or dessert item first.

- Buy tubes of cake decorator gel or glucose gel (a product designed for people with diabetes). These products are easy for someone else to squeeze into your mouth if hypoglycemia makes you confused or combative. Instruct family and friends that they should never force any form of sugar or gel into your mouth if you are unconscious: You could choke or inhale the substance into your lungs.

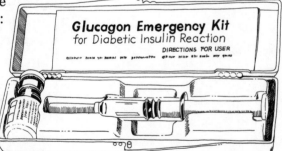

- Tell friends or family to ask you a question that requires you to think or problem-solve if they suspect your blood glucose is low. Asking if you are OK is not enough to make an accurate judgment of your condition.

If signs and symptoms are not treated, a severe episode of hypoglycemia can occur. Treatment for severe hypoglycemia is 1 milligram (mg) of Glucagon for adults and 0.5 mg for children younger than six years of age. The Glucagon kit has glucose and water, which is mixed and injected with a syringe. Glucagon is not intended as a self-treatment. It is used to treat someone who is unable to swallow or is unconscious. Store your Glucagon kit in the refrigerator. Be sure family and friends know where it is and how to use it.

ADJUST YOUR INSULIN.

Research has shown that adjusting insulin based on blood glucose values can improve diabetes control. You learn to anticipate how much insulin you need for various activities and foods. This practice is particularly effective for those who require multiple injections or an insulin pump, but it also works for people who take two injections a day. Your diabetes educator can help you evaluate patterns (described in Remedy 42) and, based on the type of insulin you use, help you adjust your dose.

Insulin is derived from various sources. Human insulin is the most common. Despite what its name suggests, human insulin does not come from humans; it is manufactured synthetically in a laboratory. Its structure is identical to insulin the body produces. Purified animal insulin, such as pork and beef, is also available. These insulins have a somewhat longer duration of action than human insulin.

Insulin	Begins to Work	Peaks	Duration
Rapid-Acting (Regular)	½–1 hour	2–4 hours	5–8 hours
Intermediate-Acting (NPH, Lente)	1–4 hours	6–10 hours	10–14 hours
Long-Acting (Ultralente)	4–6 hours	12–18 hours	24 hours
Premixed, mixture of intermediate- and short-acting (70/30, 50/50)	½–1 hour	2–12 hours	22–24 hours

It is easiest to make changes in Regular insulin: Because it works over a shorter time span, your adjustments can be more precise. You can adjust the dose to compensate for a high or low blood glucose, more or less food, or exercise. If you're considering adjusting your insulin regimen, follow this advice:

- Check with your doctor or diabetes educator first. Don't adjust your insulin without their support and recommendations.

- It is generally safe to make changes within 10 percent of the usual dose of insulin. For example, if you normally take 20 units of NPH, a change of 2 units in either direction is generally acceptable.

- Don't make daily changes in your NPH, Lente, or Ultralente insulin unless directed to do so. It usually takes about three days to see the effect of a dose adjustment of these insulins. Also wait to see a pattern of high blood glucose results before increasing these insulins. Don't increase the dose based on one high result.

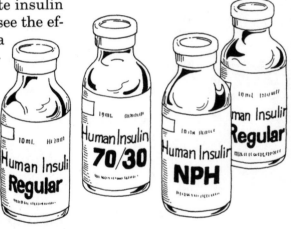

- If you have an unexplained low blood glucose result, don't wait for another one before making an adjustment to prevent it. In other words, if you didn't eat enough or you got more exercise than usual, don't adjust your insulin; you know what caused the problem and can fix it the next time. But if you ate normally, took your usual amount of insulin, had your usual amount of exercise, but your blood glucose was still low, reduce the amount of insulin by 10 percent.

- If your glucose results fall into a pattern of high/low/high/low, don't continue to increase insulin to get the high numbers down. You may be experiencing a rebound effect (see Remedy 42); each time you increase insulin to cover the high numbers, you will likely cause low blood glucose, and the bouncing will continue. Talk to your doctor or diabetes educator—you may actually need to decrease the amount of insulin.

38 WATCH FOR KETONES.

Normally, the body uses glucose to feed its cells, which need the sugar for energy to function. When not enough insulin is available to help glucose reach the cells, a process begins whereby stored fat is changed to energy to try to feed the starving cells. One of the by-products of fat breakdown is ketones. Think of ketones like ashes in a fireplace: When you burn a log in the fire, ashes are left. When you burn fat, ketones are left.

Ketones build up in the blood and spill into the urine. They pull water from the blood into the urine, causing dehydration. They can also lead to a very serious condition called ketoacidosis. Ketoacidosis can develop over a period of days or very suddenly with a virus or vomiting illness. Untreated ketoacidosis can progress to a coma. Signs of ketoacidosis are: fruity-smelling breath; labored breathing; nausea, vomiting, stomach pain; dry, flushed skin; dehydration (sunken eyes, cracked lips, dry mouth); lethargy, drowsiness.

Ketones develop as a result of insufficient insulin, not, as some people mistakenly believe, from eating too much food or too many sweets.

Pharmacies carry strips to test your urine for ketones. You simply pass a strip through your urine stream and compare the color of the strip with a color chart on the bottle. If you have ketones, consult your doctor or diabetes educator right away. If you have both ketones in your urine and high blood glucose levels, your doctor may recommend more insulin.

- Test urine for ketones when you are sick. This is particularly important if you have a fever or are vomiting.

- Test for ketones any time you have a single blood glucose result higher than 300 mg/dL or a level that remains higher than 240 mg/dL for more than a day.

- If you have ketones, drink sugar-free soda or powdered drinks in addition to water because you need to replace sodium and potassium.

TRY TURNING UP THE INTENSITY.

Have you considered intensive insulin therapy? This treatment involves multiple daily injections of insulin or use of an insulin pump. Its aim is to give you tighter control and more flexibility at the same time. Seem hard to believe? Read on.

With multiple daily injections, you add to the number of injections you currently take. If you now take one injection of insulin, try two and see what effect it has on your blood glucose level. Additional injections can be worth the extra effort if they normalize your blood glucose levels and prevent or delay the complications of diabetes. You will feel better, too! If you now require two injections, you might do better with three or even four! What have you got to lose by trying? True, you may find multiple daily injections just don't work well for you. Or you may decide they aren't worth the effort. On the other hand, this method may improve your blood glucose levels and add some flexibility to your diabetes management.

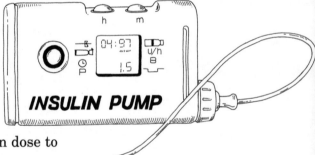

INSULIN PUMP

The use of multiple daily injections allows you to have a more varied schedule or to eat and drink more spontaneously. Here's how it works. You take a long-acting insulin once or twice a day and Regular insulin before meals and, sometimes, snacks. You can decide before you eat what you'll eat and change the insulin dose to match. If you want to eat less, you take less insulin. If you want to eat more, or you have a high blood glucose level, you take more insulin. Clearly, this treatment method allows you more flexibility. If you don't take insulin before lunch currently, you must be more careful about controlling your midday meal content and portions. In fact, you actually have to know what you are going to have for lunch when you take your injection at breakfast.

An insulin pump can also give you this flexibility. You clip the pump to a belt, bra, or waistband, or keep it in a pocket. The pump, about the size of a pager, holds a syringe that contains Regular (short-acting) insulin.

The syringe is connected to a fine tubing with an ultrafine needle at the end, which you insert into the fatty tissue of your abdomen and tape down. The needle stays taped in place until you change the spot in a few days (to avoid infections). A little bit of Regular insulin is pumped in all day long. This is called the basal amount of insulin, or the insulin your body needs between meals. You can program your pump to give you different amounts of basal insulin based on your need. For example, you may require about 1 unit of insulin per hour throughout most of the day but only ½ unit per hour in the evening because you are very active with your children. Before meals and snacks, you program your pump to give you a dose of insulin to balance the amount of food you will eat.

When you use multiple daily injection or pump therapy, you must test blood glucose four times a day; usually before meals and bedtime and once a week during the night. You base your insulin doses on your current blood glucose and the foods you plan to eat. If you're considering intensive insulin therapy, here's some advice:

- Give it at least a month trial before you decide if this treatment is right for you. It usually takes several weeks to become regulated and several more to get the gist of fine-tuning control. The companies that manufacture pumps give you 30 days to try a pump, so you don't have to commit to the purchase before you know if you like it.

- Discuss the pros and cons of each method with others who use intensive insulin therapy.

- Discuss the use of an insulin pump with your partner. Your partner may have concerns about whether the pump will affect your level of intimacy. There is little danger of the needle dislodging; however, if this is a fear, you can disconnect the pump for short periods of time. Just make sure you don't fall asleep without reconnecting the pump!

- Practice wearing a pump using an infusion set filled with saline instead of insulin for a few days. You can find out what it feels like to have the needle inserted and the pump attached.

STORE YOUR INSULIN PROPERLY.

Insulin is a protein, and proteins are sensitive to extremes in temperature. If insulin freezes or overheats, it breaks down and does not work properly. Follow this advice to ensure that your insulin stays in its proper form.

- Insulin is stable at room temperature for at least one month, so you can carry it in your pocket, purse, or briefcase. Just protect it from intense heat, direct sunlight, and freezing cold; in other words, don't leave it in the car or on a windowsill! Other unsuitable storage spots are the top of the refrigerator and the bathroom medicine cabinet.

- For travel in hot weather, pack insulin in a cooler.

- Store extra insulin in the refrigerator. An area of the refrigerator that does not freeze, such as the butter keeper, is an ideal place to keep it. Keep insulin in its box to keep the bottle clean and shield the contents from the light.

- Consider warming insulin to room temperature before administering a dose. Doing so may make the injection more comfortable. It also allows the insulin to work within its time frame because it doesn't have to take as long to warm up to body temperature. Although insulin manufacturers recommend that insulin be kept cool, insulin loses only about 1.5 percent of its potency over 30 days at room temperature, an amount not noticeable enough to make a difference in control.

- If you use NPH, Lente, or Ultralente insulin, roll the bottle between your palms or tip it gently from top to bottom to mix it before drawing it into the syringe. The cloudy appearance of these types of insulin identifies them as suspensions, which means their particles may settle during storage and must be mixed with the liquid before each use.

- If you notice a frosting on the sides of the bottles or if the insulin clumps in the bottle, do not use the insulin.

- Do not use insulin after the expiration date printed on the vial label and the carton.

- If a change occurs in your blood glucose control and you can't think of a reason for it, switch to a new bottle of insulin to see if your glucose results improve.

- When you travel by air, bring insulin in carry-on baggage. Don't worry about passing through security as the airport scanning machines will not harm insulin.

- If you need to fill syringes ahead of time, keep them refrigerated and use them within 21 days. Don't forget to roll or tip prefilled syringes that contain longer-acting insulin preparations before injecting the insulin.

- Try an insulin pen. The pen holds a cartridge of 150 units of insulin. You simply dial the proper dose instead of drawing it up in a syringe.

BE PREPARED!

Diabetes care is one area of your life where you really don't want surprises. So use a bit of forethought to help you stay in control.

• Inventory necessary supplies regularly, perhaps on the first of each month. Don't let supplies get too low. You don't want to run out when pharmacies are closed or find that your pharmacy must special order your prescription.

• If you take insulin, keep at least one extra bottle of each kind of insulin on hand. If you break a bottle or something else happens to it, your backup will save you an urgent trip to the pharmacy.

• If you take NPH or Lente insulin only, ask your doctor if it is worthwhile to keep a bottle of Regular (short-acting) insulin on hand for use in special situations when your blood glucose level is high such as during illness. See Remedy 37 for a discussion of the time-action curves of different types of insulin.

• Check your meter case regularly to make sure you have enough strips and lancets. Make sure the meter's code matches the code on the bottle of strips. Keep an extra supply of batteries on hand if your meter is battery-operated. Don't forget to check your second meter, too, if you have one that you keep at work or carry with you!

• When you travel, pack twice as many supplies as you think you will use (see Remedy 49).

• If you are hiking, boating, or are otherwise away from people and food, pack far more food and glucose tablets than you think you will need, especially if you take insulin. Also pack your Glucagon kit and show someone how to use it.

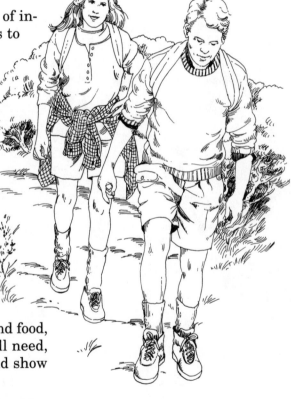

• Always have some readily available form of sugar with you. Keep extra crackers and juice boxes in the car to treat hypoglycemia and a six-pack of diet soda in case it's not available where you're going.

• Always wear a medical ID (see Remedy 33).

42 LOOK FOR PATTERNS.

Learning to identify patterns in your diabetes control is a valuable tool. It takes practice and it takes diligence, but the results are well worth it. Your doctor and diabetes educator will want to see your daily medication, blood glucose, and food records, and they'll help you learn to evaluate them yourself. If you control diabetes by means of diet and exercise, watching for patterns is less critical but still useful. It allows you to see how your blood glucose responds to certain foods and different types of exercise.

To detect patterns of control, you must first have a good understanding of your medication. If you require an oral agent or insulin, know the name of the medication, when it begins to work, when it works the hardest (when the action peaks), and how long it works.

Record periods of activity, exercise, or stress as well as foods and eating patterns. If you had extra food one day or a special treat, write it down. Likewise, it's important to know if you missed a meal, ate lightly, or were sick. Here are some other ideas to help you study your patterns.

- Recognize that two heads are better than one. Study your records with a family member or friend. He or she can help you remember that a particular entry coincides with the night you went to the mall or went bike riding.

- Use color to help you keep track. Purchase two different-colored highlighter markers. Highlight low numbers (less than your target range) in, say, yellow and high numbers (greater than your target range) in pink. After a couple of weeks, study the pattern. When are the highs and lows occurring? Why do you think they occur when they do? If your page looks very "pink" at supper, can you determine why you consistently run over your target range then? Have you been snacking too much in the afternoon? Are certain foods to blame? Are you eating a large midday meal? Or are you eating appropriately, which means you may need an adjustment in your medications or exercise schedule?

- Compare bedtime readings with your dinner menu. Can you track high bedtime readings to certain foods? For example, do you notice that blood glucose levels are particularly high when you eat spaghetti, Mexican food, or mashed potatoes? If you take pills, you might want to experiment by eating less of the foods you suspect cause glucose levels to rise, or exercise longer before or after that meal. If you take insulin, ask your doctor or educator if he or she suggests you take extra insulin on nights you eat these foods.

- Recognize that all foods are not created equal. Some are more refined and as a result more easily absorbed than others. Some have more fat, resulting in a slower rate of absorption. (The effects of a particular food may even vary greatly from one person to the next.) Figure these facts into your control. If you notice a toasted oats cereal causes a greater rise than cornflakes, choose the toasted oats on an active morning and choose the cornflakes on a less hectic morning.

- Look for a pattern of low blood glucose after exercise. If such a pattern occurs, how long after exercise does it occur? Are blood glucose levels too low in the morning when you exercise the evening before? If so, consider eating a little extra at bedtime, or talk to your educator or doctor about changing your diet, medication dose, or medication timing.

- Look for a pattern of high blood glucose after low results. This effect is commonly called a rebound, or Somogyi, effect; it occurs when hormones kick in to raise blood glucose when it is too low. Because the hormones continue to work for a while after blood glucose returns to normal, a high blood glucose level often follows. On the other hand, high blood glucose levels that occur after low ones may also be due to overeating or anxiety eating. Evaluating patterns helps you identify the difference.

- Keep a record of where you inject insulin. Some people notice differences in their glucose levels when they inject insulin in their arm compared with days they use their leg or abdomen.

- Look for bumps at your injection sites. Called hypertrophies, these raised areas may appear if you give your injections in the same places for a long time. They act like sponges, soaking up the insulin and preventing it from getting into the body at its usual rate.

43

MEASURE SUCCESS.

One of the ways you and your doctor will evaluate the success of your diabetes control is to review the results you obtain when you test your blood on your meter. Discuss with your doctor your target range for blood glucose levels. If your results generally run outside this target range, your doctor, diabetes educator, or registered dietitian can help you adjust your food, exercise, or medication.

Another way to assess diabetes control is with a blood test called hemoglobin A_{1C} (HbA_{1C}). Hemoglobin is a part of your red blood cells. Researchers discovered that glucose sticks to hemoglobin. The HbA_{1C} test measures the amount of glucose that stuck to the hemoglobin; this is an excellent reflection of average blood glucose control over the past two to three months.

Most people with diabetes undergo an HbA_{1C} test every three months. In general, the closer the result is to normal—so long as you don't also experience hypoglycemia—the better. Every little bit you can decrease HbA_{1C} levels helps reduce complications of diabetes.

Keep track of your HbA_{1C} results just as you do your other tests:

- Ask your doctor what your goal is for HbA_{1C} results.

- Don't compare numbers done in different laboratories or hospitals. Laboratories can use different testing methods, so make sure you know what the normal value is for the laboratory you go to most often.

- Don't be too upset if your HbA_{1C} result doesn't improve very quickly. It takes months to see significant changes.

- Evaluate your HbA_{1C} results in conjunction with your meter test results. If the HbA_{1C} value is high, indicating a high average blood glucose, and your meter numbers are normal, something is amiss. It could be a problem with your meter accuracy, or you may be testing blood glucose only at times your blood glucose is within normal range. On the other hand, if your HbA_{1C} value is reasonable and your meter results are high, you know that good control is within reach.

DO WHAT IT TAKES!

It's easy to be complacent with diabetes care, pushing it on the back burner as other concerns—house, kids, family, school, friends, work, and so on—take priority. But diabetes care needs to be important enough in your life so you continue to do the very best you can to care for yourself. Why settle for less?

What's more, your diabetes program should be dynamic, changing with your individual needs and the progress new technology and new research bring. Consequently, you probably will not follow the same management program for the rest of your life. Gone are the days when a person took one unchanging dose of insulin for 30 years. And unless you are in perfect control right now (not many people fall into that category), most assuredly you can take steps to improve your level of control.

If what you are doing currently does not give you optimal diabetes control, with your doctor's direction, move to the next level of control:

- If you are on a diet and exercise program, consider taking an oral agent.

- If you take an oral agent, your doctor may want to change your dose or try another agent.

- If you have reached the maximum dose with oral agents and blood glucose levels remain higher than your target range, you may need to take insulin.

- If you are currently on NPH or Lente insulin alone, you may need to add Regular insulin or switch to a premixed insulin.

- If you require one injection currently, you may need to increase to two.

- If you require two injections currently, you may do better with multiple daily injections.

- If you take multiple daily injections currently, you may do well on an insulin pump (see Remedy 37).

COVER YOURSELF.

There is no question that diabetes is an expensive disease. And negotiating the insurance scene can be complicated and confusing. In fact, do you really understand your health benefits? Obviously, the purpose of health insurance is to save out-of-pocket expenses for health care. But to ensure you receive all the benefits you're entitled to so you don't spend more than you should, you must understand the finer points of your insurance coverage.

- Does the plan allow referral to an endocrinologist, or must you be treated by your primary care physician?

- How many physician and education visits does the plan cover?

- Do you have coverage for diabetes education, including nutrition education? In some states, insurance companies provide coverage for diabetes education if the program has been recognized by the American Diabetes Association or the State Department of Health as meeting certain standards of care and education.

- Does your plan specify what type of meter you can purchase? Does it cover the cost of testing strips? Strips, which average about 60 cents each, can add up to a major expense.

- If your insurance does not cover expenses for preventive diabetes care, consider submitting a letter of medical necessity for services and supplies to encourage the insurance company to cover these costs. Sometimes a physician's letter or support of the cost-effectiveness of diabetes education from your educator can supply insurance companies with rationale for providing the coverage you need. A copy of this letter should also be given to your employee benefits personnel so your employer can also encourage the insurance company to supply coverage of diabetes care.

Talk with your insurance agent or employee benefits representative if you have any questions. And follow this advice for coping with the paperwork:

- Make sure you file your claims to the proper portion of your benefit plan; most plans have basic and supplemental portions.

- Try not to file a claim until your expenses exceed your yearly deductible, but don't delay filing. Generally, claims must be filed by the end of the calendar year following the year the charges were incurred.

- Submit itemized bills. Balance due, paid on account, and cash register receipts may not be acceptable. Bills should include the name and address of the provider, patient's full name, date of service, description of services performed, amount charged for each service, and the diagnosis.

- Keep copies of your submissions for your files.

- If your coverage includes a prescription plan, learn how prescriptions should be written. For example, some plans cover a three-month supply of medication, and prescriptions must be written that way. Other plans request that all medications be written on one prescription. Know what your plan requires, and ask your doctor's office to place this information in your records so you will not endure a delay when you need supplies.

If you're considering switching to a new plan or policy, be sure to find out if any new plan contains a preexisting illness clause that either excludes coverage of diabetes care completely or excludes care for a certain waiting period (such as six months to a year). Be truthful when you fill out insurance applications. Misrepresentation can lead to cancellation of your policy and denial of benefits.

If you apply for coverage and are denied, provide evidence that diabetes is well controlled and that you are either free of complications or they are stabilized. Your doctor can help by submitting a letter with laboratory results confirming good control. You should also inquire about state services for people with diabetes. Many states now have "pooled risk" insurance plans for people who have difficulty getting group coverage. The premiums for these plans may be a bit higher than others, but you can purchase comprehensive health insurance at an affordable cost. Contact the Office of the Insurance Commissioner in your state. Consider reducing your premium costs by choosing higher deductibles.

GET INVOLVED!

One way to help yourself is to get involved in diabetes organizations. Your participation in these groups helps in a couple of ways. First, you meet others with some of the same problems and concerns you have. You learn from each other's experiences. You problem-solve together. You learn that you are not the only one who feels as you do or has been through what you've been through. You may even make lifelong friendships.

Second, you play a role in helping these organizations achieve their mission and goals. Whether your interest or talent lies in fund-raising activities, bookkeeping, lobbying legislators, publicity, accounting, organizing educational programs, or just envelope-licking, you can find an organization that needs your help. And while you work with others for a common cause, you can have some fun at the same time.

You learn a lot along the way, too, by attending educational programs or seminars, reading newsletters and journals, and keeping up with current research. Because you are well informed, you make better decisions about your own care. The health professionals and people with diabetes you meet help keep you motivated.

Finally, people who have participated in diabetes organizations, fighting for research dollars, for example, are the reason diabetes care is as good as it is today. If you're interested in getting involved with a diabetes organization, contact the American Diabetes Association (1-800-232-3472) or the Juvenile Diabetes Foundation International (1-800-223-1138) for more information. Keep in mind that if diabetes organizations don't fit your bill, there are many other good causes to get involved in.

ADVOCATE FOR YOUR NEEDS ON THE JOB.

Have you ever felt discriminated against in the workplace because you have diabetes? If an employer has ever refused to allow you time to take insulin or test your blood, to eat meals or snacks, or to store necessary diabetes supplies in your work area, you know what it's like to be made to feel different as a result of a medical condition or made to feel as if your condition makes you somehow less competent in the workplace.

Now people with diabetes and other medical conditions have support. Diabetes is considered a disability under the Americans with Disabilities Act of 1990. The purpose of the Act is to eliminate discrimination against people with disabilities; it became effective in July 1992 for employers with 25 or more employees and July 1994 for employers with 15 or more employees. The act ensures equal employment opportunities for people with disabilities. In addition, it states that "reasonable accommodation" must be made for persons with disabilities. Reasonable accommodation includes making existing facilities accessible to employees with disabilities; restructuring a job; modifying the work schedule; acquiring new or modifying existing equipment or devices; and modifying examinations, training materials, or policies to make them appropriate for individuals with disabilities. The employer, however, need not provide accommodation if doing so would be significantly difficult or expensive (it would incur "undue hardship"). The Equal Employment Opportunity Commission (EEOC) investigates complaints of violations of the Act.

The Act protects your rights in the workplace. You can help by observing these tips for managing diabetes in the workplace.

- Make sure someone knows you have diabetes. Your condition does not need to be public information, but someone—a supervisor or coworker—

should know you have diabetes, how you treat it, and where you keep your supplies.

- Tell your employer what you need to manage diabetes. If you need to eat a snack or take your lunch at a certain time, for example, let your employer know this. Most employers try to be accommodating.

- If altering a work schedule proves difficult or problematic, you may be able to change your diabetes management schedule. For example, if taking lunch at noon is not possible or desirable (maybe the lunch hour is the busiest time of day at your job), you may be able to adjust your insulin or add a snack in the morning.

- If possible, keep your diabetes supplies in a desk drawer or somewhere close to your work site. If you need to test during the day, you may be able to test quickly and inconspicuously at your desk and get on with your work.

- If you believe you are being discriminated against because you have diabetes, call the Equal Employment Opportunity Commission office at 1-800-669-4000.

DRIVE SAFELY.

When hypoglycemia (low blood glucose) occurs, the brain, deprived of glucose, cannot function properly. Clouded judgment, impaired reaction time, confusion, and disorientation can result. Obviously, this is not a good state to be in while driving, for you or for anyone else on the road.

Take precautions before you get behind the wheel:

- Always test your blood glucose level before you drive. Carry testing equipment with you.

- Always carry a form of fast-acting sugar as well as a follow-up snack containing protein! Keep extras handy for unexpected events such as when you're caught in rush hour traffic or the car breaks down. Store peanut butter crackers, juice boxes, and glucose tablets in the glove compartment. And don't forget to replace any food supplies you use!

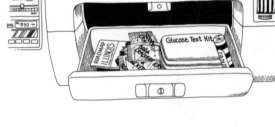

- If you experience hypoglycemia symptoms, pull off the road and wait until your blood glucose level returns to normal range and your symptoms have ended before continuing.

- Drive with a companion when possible.

- If you are the driver on a long trip, you may reduce your calories by 100 the day(s) you are in the car. When you hit big-city traffic, make sure you have an extra snack to protect yourself from low blood glucose that could result from stress.

- Stop to test your blood glucose at 3- to 4-hour intervals or any time you suspect hypoglycemia.

Don't leave insulin unprotected in your vehicle while you're sightseeing or dining, especially on a very hot or cold day. A change in the potency could occur even though the insulin may not look any different. Use a thermos or insulated travel pack to store insulin safely.

Follow appropriate precautions when you operate other types of motor vehicles, such as boats, tractors, and snowmobiles.

49 | PACK FOR TRAVEL.

Clutching your plane ticket and itinerary, you smile when you think about how much you're going to enjoy this trip. But the smile fades when you realize that for all your careful planning, you've forgotten to plan how to fit diabetes control into this vacation. How will you handle the change in time zones? Will you be able to find appropriate foods at your destination? You place a call to your diabetes educator, who confirms that travel can present some challenges but assures you that diabetes care is generally available worldwide. Your educator points out that if you follow some commonsense tips for travel, you should be able to hit the road without hitting too many snags. Start with what you pack:

- Take plenty of supplies. Double the amount you anticipate you'll need in the event of any problems. Insulin bottles can break, and replacing them may not be easy. If you do break a bottle of insulin, go to a local pharmacy or emergency room for insulin. If the country you're visiting has another strength of insulin (U-40 or U-80), also purchase syringes to match so you measure the dose accurately.

- Keep your supplies with you at all times. If you're flying, place your meter, strips, insulin, syringes, and snacks or glucose tablets in carry-on luggage, not in your check-in baggage. If you need them during the flight, it's usually a good idea to explain briefly to the person sitting next to you what you're doing with that needle. In general, people are supportive and will probably tell you about their friends and family members with diabetes. Pack enough food in carry-on bags to replace the carbohydrates you might normally consume at a meal. Crackers and raisins are easy to transport.

- Keep insulin in an insulated container, especially if you're traveling to a warm climate. A wide-mouth thermos works well for this. Travel packs designed for this purpose are available.

- If you're hiking, biking, mountain climbing, or boating, carry plenty of food and a fast-acting source of sugar. If you have a problem with severe hypoglycemia, take a Glucagon kit along, and teach someone how and when to use it. Keep your meter with you, too.

- Travel with a buddy, if possible, and ask him or her to carry extra supplies for you as well. If you're traveling alone, make sure your carry-on bag or briefcase is well stocked.

- Take sugar-free powdered drink mix if you're traveling to a country where diet drinks are not readily available. Mix it with bottled water.

- When traveling outside the United States, obtain a prescription from your doctor, stating that you have diabetes and that you are required to carry syringes. Wear your medical ID to show customs personnel in case you are questioned.

Crossing time zones can really throw your management schedule off. Depending on the distance you travel, you could lose or gain as much as a day. Your diabetes educator can help you plot out your home schedule and that of your destination to see how the time differences will affect your usual eating and medication times.

- If you're flying, call the airlines to ask when food is usually served. Airlines prepare special meals if you request them 24 hours ahead of time.

- Keep your watch on home time until you arrive at your destination. This allows you to adjust your schedule correctly in the new time zone. Or purchase a traveler's watch with two faces.

Ask your registered dietitian for advice on adjusting to different types of foods. In some countries, meats, fresh fruits, or vegetables may be a rarity; diets may consist of a lot of complex carbohydrates, such as beans, corn, bread, and rice. You'll need to adjust your medication accordingly. Also, if beer or wine is the culture's beverage of choice at mealtimes, you'll need to calculate these extra calories into your plan. The evening meal in Spanish-speaking countries is typically quite late. Consider reversing your bedtime snack and evening meal to accommodate this habit, or take more Regular insulin at the late meal and less NPH insulin.

If you travel frequently, you might consider a more flexible regimen such as an insulin pump or multiple daily injections.

LEARN THE LINGO

If you cannot speak the language of the country you're visiting, at least learn these few critical phrases:

"I have diabetes."

"I need sugar or orange juice."

"Please get me a doctor."

The International Association for Medical Assistance to Travelers has centers in 125 countries with English- or French-speaking physicians who are on call 24 hours a day.

50

CARPE DIEM: SEIZE THE DAY!

Don't let diabetes become an excuse. Don't let it keep you from doing what you should and want to do. Yes, taking care of diabetes requires time, energy, and lots of focus. But once you learn to fit diabetes into your lifestyle, it should not get in the way of activities you really want to pursue. In fact, diabetes can give you a heightened appreciation of your health and the strong desire to keep it. It may lead you to see how precious every moment is.

Living with diabetes can also help you keep your priorities straight. We all have responsibilities and commitments. But too many of us spend what little free time we have worrying about problems we can't solve and performing activities we don't find fulfilling. Make time for activities you enjoy! It is not selfish to do what makes you feel happy and fulfilled. Taking care of yourself, preserving your health, and seeking satisfaction in daily life are the best gifts you can give to those you care about and those who care about you. Do what you need and want to do. And take care of diabetes along the way.

INDEX

Hypertension, 26, 27, 34, 35, 36, 41, 46
Hypertrophies, 67
Hypoglycemia, 56–57, 68
  prevention of, 8, 36, 47, 48, 65, 75
  symptoms and treatment, 14, 15, 22, 23, 25, 26, 36, 42, 56–57, 75

Identification, medical, 51, 65
Illness, effect on diabetes, 18, 22, 25, 42–43, 66
Impotence, 52
Infections, 21, 39, 44, 45, 53
Insulin
  adjusting doses, 22, 26, 28, 36, 37, 38, 42, 55, 58–59, 62, 69
  peak action and duration, 18, 22, 23, 26, 37, 66
  storage, 63–64, 75, 76
  types, 55, 58–59, 63
Insulin infusion pump, 6, 19, 22, 37, 58, 61–62, 69, 77
Insulin injection, methods, 20, 23–24, 41, 63, 67
Insurance, health, 70–71
Intensive insulin therapy, 6, 19, 22, 37, 54–55, 58, 61–62, 69, 77
Intimacy, 5, 62. *See also* Sexual function.
Juvenile Diabetes Foundation International, 13, 15, 72

Juvenile-onset diabetes. *See* Type I diabetes.

Ketoacidosis, 60
Ketones, 22, 26, 42, 43, 55, 60
Kidney disease, 5, 6, 7, 34, 35

Lancets, 8, 17, 21

Meal planning, 5, 6, 9, 14, 15, 18, 22, 25, 27–38, 45, 55, 77
Medications, for diabetes, 8, 14, 15, 18, 19, 20, 22, 23, 36, 37, 42, 45, 55, 56, 66, 69
Menstruation, 52–53
Meters, 8, 16, 25, 41, 65, 68, 70, 76
Motivation, 6, 7
Multiple daily injections. *See* Intensive insulin therapy.

Nephropathy, 5
Nervous system, 6, 35, 36, 48, 52, 53. *See also* Neuropathy.
Neuropathy, 5, 35, 39, 40
Non–insulin-dependent diabetes, 5

Ophthalmologist, 41
Oral health, 44–45

Periodontitis, 44
Positive outlook, 6, 12, 49
Pregnancy, 53, 54–55

Rebound effect, 59, 67
Record keeping, 12, 18, 19, 25, 28, 55
Relaxation techniques, 48–49
Retinopathy, 5, 41, 54

Salt. *See* Sodium.
Schedule, keeping a, 14, 19–20, 26, 28, 37, 38, 66, 67
Sexual function, 52–53
Smoking, 12, 39, 46, 55
Sodium, 32, 34
Somogyi effect. *See* Rebound effect.
Starch. *See* Carbohydrates.
Stress, 9, 18, 42, 48–49, 52, 66, 75
Sugar, 26, 32, 39, 44, 53, 75, 76. *See also* Carbohydrates; Hypoglycemia, symptoms and treatment.
Supplements, dietary, 35
Syringes, 8, 17, 23, 24, 64, 76

Travel, 63, 64, 65, 76–77
Type I diabetes, 5, 7, 19, 39
Type II diabetes, 5, 19, 39

Vascular system, 39, 40, 46, 52

Weight and weight control, 5, 12, 15, 28, 32, 52